Education Standards
for
Critical Care Nursing

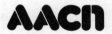

Education Standards *for* Critical Care Nursing

American Association of Critical-Care Nurses

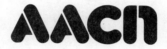

THE C. V. MOSBY COMPANY

St. Louis • Toronto • Princeton   1986

MOSBY

A TRADITION OF PUBLISHING EXCELLENCE

Editor: David P. Carroll
Assistant editor: Sharon Haegele
Cover design: Susan Lane

Top Graphics
Project manager: Billie Forshee
Manuscript editor: Connie Leinicke
Book design: Susan Trail
Production: Susan Trail

International Standard Book Number 0-8016-0156-8

Printed in the United States of America

The C.V. Mosby Company
11830 Westline Industrial Drive, St. Louis, Missouri 63146

AC/VH/VH 9 8 7 6 5 4 3 2 1   01/D/083

—Education Standards Task Force

Editor-in-Chief:

JoAnn Grif Alspach, RN, MSN, CCRN
Editor, *Critical Care Nurse,*
Consultant, Critical Care Nursing
    Education, Annapolis, Maryland

Editors:

Judith Bell, RN, EdD
Medical Clinical Specialist,
Veterans Administration Hospital,
Omaha, Nebraska

Mary M. Canobbio, RN, MN
Cardiovascular Clinical Specialist,
Division of Cardiology,
Assistant Clinical Professor,
School of Nursing,
University of California Los Angeles,
Los Angeles, California

Susan B. Christoph, RN, DNSc, CCRN
Chief Nurse,
U.S. Army Medical Research and
    Development Command,
Fort Dietrich,
Frederick, Maryland

Rebecca C. Kuhn, RN, MS, CCRN
Critical Care Clinical Specialist,
St. Luke's Hospital,
Phoenix, Arizona

Wanda L. Roberts, RN, MN, CCRN
Director of Critical Care Nursing,
Overlake Hospital Medical Center,
Bellevue, Washington

Lane Turzan, RN, MN
Associate Director of Education,
Continuing Education Review-Standards,
American Association of Critical-Care
    Nurses,
Newport Beach, California

Clareen Wiencek, RN, MSN, CCRN
Formerly Unit Director for Medical
    Intensive Care Units,
Indiana University Hospital,
Indiana University Medical Center,
Indianapolis, Indiana

___ Preface

In the Spring of 1981, the AACN Board of Directors directed that a task force be established to develop the *Education Standards for Critical Care Nursing.* Over the next four years, members of the task force responded to this challenge by providing the documents that comprise this book.

A number of assumptions guided development of this project:

- That the AACN *Education Standards for Critical Care Nursing* should be consistent with existing AACN policies, procedures, goals, position statements, and other organizational pronouncements;
- That the *Education Standards for Critical Care Nursing* should be consistent with the AACN *Standards for Nursing Care of the Critically Ill*[1];
- That critical care nursing education is "education directed at facilitating application of the knowledge, skills, and attitudes required for competent critical care nursing practice."[2] In this regard, critical care nursing education is a *means* to an end rather than an end in itself. Only when the critical care nurse integrates and applies this knowledge, as well as these attitudes and skills, can optimal nursing care of the critically ill be achieved.
- That as a professional and as an adult learner, the individual nurse is ultimately responsible for the learning necessary to maintain competency and currency in critical care nursing practice.
- That insofar as possible, the *Education Standards* should be consistent with related sets of standards and terminology used throughout the nursing profession.

The components of this project include the following:

1. Conceptual Framework for the *Education Standards for Critical Care Nursing.* This framework was constructed to ensure consistency of the *Education Standards* with other AACN organizational positions and statements and to establish a foundation for deriving, implementing, and evaluating the *Education Standards.* This document contains the conceptual *model* for the project, a graphic illustration of how

---

[1] American Association of Critical-Care Nurses: *Standards for nursing care of the critically ill,* Reston, Va., 1981, Reston Publishing Co.
[2] Alspach, J.G.: *Issues in critical care education.* Keynote address. Presented at AACN Leadership Institute, Chicago, 1983.

the *Education Standards* relate to AACN organizational statements, the nursing process, and the broad field of education.

2. The *Education Standards for Critical Care Nursing.* This section includes a statement of each standard, the rationale for the standard, and one or more criteria for determining compliance with the standard.

Two types of standards are used, structure and process. The *structure standards* are statements of quality that address the environment in which critical care nursing education is provided. The *process standards* are statements of quality that address actions, changes, or functions in critical care nursing education which bring about a desired end. Attainment of the *Education Standards for Critical Care Nursing* should enable the critical care nurse (learner) to meet the practice standards established for critical care nursing, that is, AACN's *Standards for Nursing Care of the Critically Ill.*

The *Education Standards for Critical Care Nursing* are collectively intended as optimal rather than minimal statements of quality. In this regard, these standards reflect ultimate expressions of quality rather than minimal expectations. The *Education Standards* should be used as guideposts in striving toward optimal levels of critical care nursing education.

A glossary is provided as an appendix to this section. The glossary offers the operational definitions of terms used in the *Education Standards.*

To maximize validity, the *Standards* statements underwent multiple drafts prior to their finalization in August 1985. Preliminary drafts of the *Standards* were sent for critique to the AACN Board of Directors and over thirty critical care nursing education providers in various settings, geographic locations, and agencies.

3. Critical Care Nursing Education: Literature Overview. The inceptual phase of this project required an extensive review of the literature related to critical care nursing education. Because this literature base had not been reported previously, the task force prepared its findings for dissemination to all critical care nurses.

The literature overview characterizes seven features of critical care nursing education as it exists in academic, service, and private settings: (1) the rationale for providing this education, (2) the individual and institutional providers, (3) how this education is provided, (4) the expected outcomes of the education, (5) the means by which this education is evaluated, (6) factors that affect this education, and (7) related sets of professional standards. The overview also identifies areas where additional research in this field is warranted.

4. Survey of Critical Care Nursing Education. A survey on the field of critical care nursing education was conducted to characterize the current state-of-the-art in this area and to afford a basis for evaluating the effect of the *Education Standards.* This book includes the analysis and final report of survey findings as described by the consulting firm that provided the survey services. The instrument used for the survey is included in Appendix B of this book. A pilot test of the survey instrument was conducted prior to its implementation.

The critical care nurses who use the *Education Standards* will provide our ultimate test of the relevancy of these statements. As the fields of critical care nursing practice and critical care nursing education evolve, we hope you will share your comments and suggestions for maintaining the relevancy of these *Standards* over time.

JoAnn Grif Alspach, RN, MSN, CCRN

Chairperson, Education Standards Task Force

___Acknowledgments

Projects such as this are accomplished through the collective efforts of dedicated professionals who contribute their time and expertise toward accomplishment of AACN goals. The *Education Standards for Critical Care Nursing* exemplify this professional commitment. The Education Standards Task Force would like to recognize Sarah Sanford, past President of AACN, for her dedication and enduring support of this project. We would also like to thank Hope Moore and Jane Petrucelli for their contributions during the formative stages of the project. We extend a deep sense of gratitude to the AACN Education Special Interest Group and the individuals and institutions who participated in the field test of the standards and the pilot test of the survey instrument. Their assistance and suggestions were invaluable to our efforts. The degree of professional staff support required for this project also merits special thanks to Lane Turzan, the Staff Liaison for the task force, and Virginia Real and Marolyn Stocker, for secretarial assistance. Our Board Liaisons, Becky Kuhn and Wanda Roberts, provided that necessary linkage between the *Education Standards* project and other AACN groups and activities.

—— Contents

— Education Standards for Critical Care Nursing: A Conceptual Framework*

The purpose of the American Association of Critical-Care Nurses (AACN) is to "promote the health and welfare of mankind by enhancing the science and art of critical care nursing."[1] One of AACN's long-range goals is to promote educational standards for critical care nursing. The *Education Standards for Critical Care Nursing* endeavors to ensure that the critical care nurse has the requisite knowledge base and clinical proficiency necessary for competency in critical care nursing.

This article presents the conceptual framework for the *Education Standards for Critical Care Nursing*. A conceptual framework is necessary to (1) ensure consistency of the *Education Standards* with the purpose, goals, and philosophy of AACN and its components and (2) establish a framework for the development, implementation, and evaluation of the *Education Standards,* thereby making underlying assumptions explicit and affording operational definitions for communication of constructs incorporated into the model.

The conceptual framework for the *Standards* arises from a conceptual model (Figure 1) composed of two major elements: the *sphere* of critical care nursing, which rests on a *base* of general education principles.

The construct of general education, which provides the foundation for the model, includes learning theory and principles of adult education. Inherent in these theories is the accountability of the individual for learning; the responsibility for learning rests with the learner. In the model, the term "education" refers to the continuing education that occurs after entry into professional nursing practice; the achievement of basic preparation in nursing is assumed.

AACN has adopted the following definition for critical care nursing: "In *Nursing: A Social Policy Statement,*[2] the American Nurses' Association defines nursing as 'the diagnosis and treatment of human responses to actual or potential health problems.' Critical care nursing is that specialty within nursing which deals specifically with

---

*Reproduced from *Heart & Lung,* March 1985, vol. 14, no. 2. Used with permission.

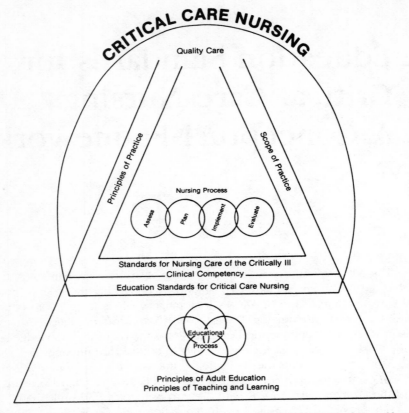

Figure 1 ── Conceptual model for the *Education Standards for Critical Care Nursing.*

human responses to life-threatening problems."[3] The sphere that encompasses critical care nursing practice envelops not only the competent practice of critical care nursing, but also the educational process facilitating attainment and maintenance of that competency. The ultimate goal of both critical care nursing and critical care nursing education is to provide quality care for critically ill patients.

The AACN Conceptual Model for Critical Care Nursing[4] deals with five major components: *Standards for Nursing Care of the Critically Ill,* AACN's Principles of Critical Care Nursing Practice, AACN's Scope of Critical Care Nursing Practice, the nursing process, and quality care.

The *Standards for Nursing Care of the Critically Ill*[5] serves as a foundation on which the remaining elements rest. The *Standards* document is a collection of structure and process standards that define quality in nursing care of critically ill patients and facilitate evaluation of the quality of care delivery. The structure standards define the physical and organizational environment in which critical care nursing is practiced. The process standards delineate critical care nursing practice. The *Standards* also direct educational efforts in staff development.

The AACN Scope of Practice Statement[6] describes critical care nursing practice as a dynamic process that is defined by three essential components: the critically ill patient, the critical care nurse, and the critical care environment.

1. The critically ill patient is "characterized by the presence of real or potential life-threatening health problems and by the requirement for continuous observation and intervention to prevent complications and restore health."

2. The critical care nurse is a registered professional nurse who is committed to providing optimal care for critically ill patients. To do so requires that the critical care nurse demonstrate the following: (a) individual professional accountability, (b) thorough knowledge of the interrelatedness of body systems and the dynamic nature of the life process, (c) recognition and appreciation of the individual's wholeness, uniqueness, and significant social and environmental relationships, and (d) appreciation of the collaborative role of all members of the health care team. Ongoing education activities ensure that competency is developed as the nurse acquires requisite knowledge and skills in the physiologic, psychosocial, and therapeutic components of care for critically ill patients.

3. The critical care environment is defined as any designated area that is equipped for the care of critically ill patients by a critical care nurse.

To further define the scope of nursing practice, AACN has issued two position statements: (1) "Integration of Critical Care Nursing Concepts and Clinical Experience Into Professional Nursing Programs,"[7] which describes the roles and responsibilities of both faculty and students in critical care settings, and (2) AACN's "Position Statement on Entry Into Practice,"[8] which states that the baccalaureate degree in nursing should be the minimal preparation for entry into professional nursing practice.

The Principles of Practice,[4] the third element of AACN's Conceptual Model for Critical Care Nursing Practice, focuses on the professional conduct of the critical care nurse. When the critical care nurse faces practice or ethical dilemmas involving nurse-patient relationships, decisions are based on underlying respect for human integrity, individuality, and rights.

The *Standards for Nursing Care of the Critically Ill,* the Scope of Practice, and the Principles of Practice form a triad within which the practice of critical care nursing occurs. Care is delivered to the patient and family through the interactive elements of the nursing process: assessment, planning, implementation, and evaluation. Utilization of the nursing process within this structure better assures a high quality of care for critically ill patients.

Effective utilization of the nursing process requires that the critical care nurse possess the requisite knowledge base and psychomotor skills for critical care nursing practice. A written certification examination and a clinical practice requirement are the two components of the AACN Certification Program. The critical care nursing content, upon which the certification examination is based, has been validated through a study[9] defining the role of the critical care nurse and delineating the requisite knowledge and skills for fulfilling this role. AACN's *Core Curriculum for Critical Care Nursing*[10] details the depth and scope of knowledge needed to practice critical care nursing.

Competent critical care nursing practice requires integration of the cognitive, psychomotor, and affective components of clinical practice and provision of nursing care consistent with the *Standards for Nursing Care of the Critically Ill,* Scope of Practice, and Principles of Practice. The outcome of clinical competency is quality care for the patient and family, which is illustrated as the apex of the model.

Competency is attained and maintained through a valid educational process. The AACN *Education Standards for Critical Care Nursing* rests on an educational framework. The educational process is dynamic and interactive and represents the foundation from which competency in critical care nursing practice develops. On a more global level, the educational process for critical care nursing derives from general education and incorporates principles of teaching and learning theory, as well as principles of adult education.

Critical care education is provided either inside or outside of the critical care environment, in academia, the service setting, and the private setting. Continuing education may occur outside of the critical care setting, while staff development activities such as orientation and in-service education are provided within the critical care environment.

Critical care nursing education is defined as "education directed at facilitating application of the knowledge, skills, and attitudes required for competent critical care nursing practice."[11] Use of the educational process, which includes assessment, planning, implementation, and evaluation, influences the practice of critical care nursing and leads to the delivery of high-quality patient care. The components of the educational process are depicted in an overlapping manner to illustrate the interactional nature of these elements.

"Educational assessment" may be defined as an organized, systematic determination of the educational needs of the critical care nurse. This assessment includes collection, organization, analysis, and validation of data related to educational needs. Assessment data are collected from a variety of sources, including the learner.

Comprehensive assessment is essential for three reasons: (1) Within each educational setting, there is a continuum of learning needs; for example, staff development in the service setting includes orientation, in-service education, and continuing education; (2) within each set of identified learning needs there is a continuum of priorities ranging from low-priority needs to high-priority needs; and (3) within any group of learners there is a continuum of abilities in cognitive, affective, and psychomotor skills. A comprehensive assessment will help facilitate individual learning.

Planning begins with prioritizing identified learning needs and delineating instructional objectives that describe expected learning outcomes. Instructional objectives provide direction for the basic structure of the program, i.e., the target audience, curriculum design, program format, faculty selection, teaching methods, resource allocation, and evaluation plan.

The implementation phase of the educational process involves execution of the educational plan. This phase is guided primarily by general principles of the teaching-learning process and adult education. While there should be consistency between the preestablished educational plan and its implementation, flexibility promotes optimal use of available resources. A support structure should facilitate maintenance of the learning environment and an adequate documentation system.

Educational evaluation validates attainment of the desired learning outcomes. Evaluation, formative and/or summative, determines the degree of effectiveness of the educational process in achieving desired outcomes. Program efficiency, as well as objectives, format, curriculum design, and administration, should be evaluated.

Institutional, professional, and individual factors, such as credentialing, and recent changes in the regulations governing health care reimbursement impinge on the educational process for critical care nursing. Existing standards related to critical care nursing may also directly or indirectly influence the provision and evaluation of critical care education.

_____ Summary

AACN exists to promote the health and welfare of mankind by advancing the science and art of critical care nursing. One of AACN's long-range goals is to promote educational standards for critical care nursing. As a prelude to dissemination of AACN's *Education Standards for Critical Care Nursing,* this article presented the conceptual framework used to develop this set of standards.

REFERENCES

1. Bylaws of the American Association of Critical-Care Nurses. Irvine, Calif., 1983, American Association of Critical-Care Nurses.
2. American Nurses' Association Congress for Nursing Practice: Nursing: a social policy statement. Kansas City, 1980, American Nurses' Association.
3. Definition of critical care nursing. Newport Beach, Calif., 1984, American Association of Critical-Care Nurses.
4. Bertram D: The concept of critical care nursing. Focus on AACN 9:5, 1982.
5. Thierer J, Perhus S, McCracken ML, Reynolds MA, Holmes AM, Turton B, Berkowitz DS, Disch JM, editors: Standards for nursing care of the critically ill. American Association of Critical-Care Nurses. Reston, Va., 1981, Reston Publishing Co.
6. Disch J: Scope of practice defined. Focus on AACN 7:18, 1980.
7. Position statement: integration of critical care nursing concepts and clinical experience into professional nursing programs. Newport Beach, Calif., 1983, American Association of Critical-Care Nurses.
8. AACN's position statement on entry into practice. Focus on AACN 8:5, 1981.
9. Role delineation study for critical care nursing. American Association of Critical-Care Nurses. Newport Beach, Calif., 1984, AACN Certification Corp.
10. Alspach JG, Williams SW, editors: Core curriculum for critical care nursing. American Association of Critical-Care Nurses. Ed. 3. Philadelphia, 1985, W.B. Saunders Co.
11. Alspach JG: Issues in critical care education. Keynote address. Presented at AACN Leadership Institute, Chicago, 1983.

___ Education Standards

___ STRUCTURE STANDARDS

1. **An administrative framework exists which facilitates provision of critical care nursing education.**

RATIONALE:

An administrative framework is necessary to ensure effective management of critical care nursing education programs.

CRITERIA:

1.1 A written philosophy exists which reflects the provider's beliefs related to critical care nursing education.

1.2 A written organizational chart exists which indicates lines of authority, responsibility, and communication.

1.3 Written policies and procedures exist for administration and management of the education program.

1.4 Documented evidence exists of educational quality assurance. This may include:
    1.41 External program review by accrediting bodies
    1.42 Internal program review based on program objectives and evaluations
    1.43 A written mechanism for and documentation of follow-up on the quality assurance outcomes
    1.44 Records of periodic performance appraisals and self-evaluations for all personnel involved in providing critical care education.

1.5 A written mechanism exists for developing a budget which reflects the financial resources necessary to implement programming.

1.6 Written position descriptions exist which identify qualifications and responsibilities for all personnel involved in critical care education.

1.7 Documentation of critical care nursing education programming exists and is readily retrievable. This documentation includes:
    1.71 Outcomes of the needs assessment
    1.72 Program planning based on identified goals
    1.73 Program budget
    1.74 Accounting of actual program revenue and expenses

1.75 Participant attendance records

1.76 Program evaluation

1.77 Evaluation of learning

1.78 Qualifications of program providers

2. Providers of critical care nursing education have the human resources to achieve program goals.

RATIONALE:

Sufficient numbers of qualified human resources are essential for attainment of critical care education program goals.

CRITERIA:

2.1 Individual providers of critical care nursing education programs meet the following qualifications:

    2.11 Competence in educational assessment, planning, implementation, and evaluation.

    2.12 Competence in the application of adult learning principles.

2.2 Support personnel are available when necessary to facilitate attainment of program goals. The staff may include, but are not limited to:

    2.21 Secretarial staff

    2.22 Audiovisual staff

    2.23 Biomedical engineer

2.3 All instructors who teach critical care nursing practice meet the following qualifications:

    2.31 A baccalaureate degree in nursing

    2.32 Knowledgeable about critical care nursing practice

    2.33 Expertise in content areas of instruction

    2.34 Competence in the application of general educational theory and adult learning principles.

2.4 Clinical nursing instructors meet the following additional qualifications:

    2.41 Meet the practice standards of the critical care unit in the area of teaching responsibility.

    2.42 Competence in assisting learners to apply concepts and principles in the care of critically ill patients.

2.5 Instructors from other health care disciplines meet the following qualifications:

    2.51 Knowledgeable in content areas of instruction.

    2.52 Competent in area of teaching responsibility.

    2.53 Competent in the application of general educational theory and adult learning principles.

2.6 The number of qualified instructors facilitates attainment of program goals.

    2.61 Criteria for the selection of instructors are consistent with the program goals.

    2.62 Instructor-learner ratios ensure patient safety.

3. Providers of critical care nursing education have the financial resources to achieve the program goals.

RATIONALE:

Achievement of program goals depends upon sound financial planning and funding of the program budget.

CRITERIA:

3.1 A mechanism exists for comparison and analysis between the program budget and actual program revenues and expenses.
3.2 A mechanism exists to relate outcomes of financial analysis to attainment of program goals.
3.3 Financial resources enable attainment of program goals.

4. Providers of critical care nursing education have the material resources to achieve program goals.

RATIONALE:

Program goals are supported by the use of material resources which enhance learning and accommodate various instructional methods and learning styles. These resources may include instructional aids such as critical care texts, reference articles, workbooks, slides, and models.

CRITERIA:

4.1 Material resources used in critical care nursing education programs are consistent with the instructional objectives.
4.2 Material resources are accurate and current.
4.3 Sufficient material resources are available to providers and participants.

5. Providers of critical care nursing education have the environmental resources to achieve program goals.

RATIONALE:

An environment conducive to learning facilitates the attainment of program goals.

CRITERIA:

5.1 Physical facilities used are consistent with the program goals and instructional objectives.
5.2 Physical facilities allow for flexibility in teaching methods, learning styles, and program scheduling.
5.3 Physical facilities are accessible to providers and participants.
5.4 Storage space is available and accessible for material resources and educational records.
5.5 Clinical experiences are available to meet instructional objectives related to nursing practice.

————— PROCESS STANDARDS

Assessment

1. **Those involved in critical care nursing education programs participate in the assessment of learning needs.**

RATIONALE:

The effectiveness of an instructional program depends upon an accurate identification of learners' educational needs. Accuracy in the identification of learning needs is increased when consideration is given to a variety of perspectives.

CRITERIA:

1.1 Learners have primary responsibility for and participate in identification of their own learning needs.
1.2 Critical care managers and instructors assist learners in identifying individual and collective learning needs.
1.3 Providers of critical care education programs facilitate the assessment process.
1.4 Individuals who participate in identifying learning needs are responsible for communicating their findings to the providers of critical care nursing education.

2. **Providers of critical care nursing education programs analyze assessment data to validate the learning needs of critical care nurses.**

RATIONALE:

A relevant curriculum depends upon an accurate delineation of learner needs and goals. Before program development is initiated, assessment data should be validated.

CRITERIA:

2.1 Providers of critical care education collect assessment data relevant to the learning needs of critical care nurses from multiple sources. These sources may include:
   2.11 Surveys, reports, questionnaires, or marketing response
   2.12 Observations of critical care nursing practice in relation to established standards of care, position descriptions, policies, procedures, and directives
   2.13 Results from quality assurance activities
   2.14 Current professional literature
   2.15 Performance appraisals
   2.16 Prior program evaluations
   2.17 Recommendations from consumers of health services

2.2   Providers assess the validity and reliability of methods used for collection of assessment data prior to data analysis.

2.3   Providers analyze assessment data relative to critical care nursing practice and the credibility of information sources.

2.4   Prior to program planning, providers of critical care nursing education programs collaborate with critical care practitioners, managers, administrators and instructors to validate conclusions drawn during the assessment process.

2.5   Providers of critical care nursing education establish priorities among learning needs relative to the philosophy and goals of the program and available resources.

3. Providers of critical care nursing education analyze resources necessary to achieve program goals as a basis for program planning.

RATIONALE:

An assessment of educational resources is necessary in the planning process. Realistic program decisions made in the planning process are influenced by the compatibility between resources and program goals.

CRITERIA:

3.1   Providers assess the following relative to program goals:

   3.11   Administrative framework
   3.12   Human resources
   3.13   Financial resources
   3.14   Material resources
   3.15   Environmental resources

4. Providers of critical care nursing education determine continued program relevance through on-going assessment of learning needs.

RATIONALE:

Learning needs change over time. An on-going assessment of learning needs in combination with program evaluation provide the basis for determining continued program relevance and the need for program revision.

CRITERIA:

4.1   Providers supply program information so that the learners can assess the congruence between their own learning needs and the goals and objectives of the educational program.

4.2   Before repeating a critical care educational program, providers verify that the established nature and priority of learning needs have remained the same.

Planning

1. **Providers of critical care nursing education use the outcomes of the assessment process to develop program goals.**

RATIONALE:

Outcomes of the needs assessment and the establishment of priorities which resulted from the assessment process serve as a basis for decision making regarding the establishment of program goals.

CRITERIA:

1.1 Program goals reflect the established priority of learning needs identified during the assessment process.

2. **Providers use program goals as a basis for developing instructional objectives.**

RATIONALE:

Program goals are needed to further specify what the learner will accomplish upon completion of the program. Instructional objectives will also provide a basis for determining attainment of program goals.

CRITERIA:

2.1 Instructional objectives are consistent with and further define the program goals.
2.2 Instructional objectives identify the cognitive, psychomotor, and/or affective behavior the learner will demonstrate following program participation.
2.3 Instructional objectives include application of knowledge and/or skills.
2.4 Instructional objectives include clearly stated and measurable performance expectations of learners.

3. **Providers design the curriculum of critical care nursing education programs on the basis of instructional objectives.**

RATIONALE:

The curriculum represents the means by which learners attain the instructional objectives.

CRITERIA:

3.1 Content of the curriculum is selected and tailored to facilitate learner attainment of the instructional objectives.
3.2 The sequence of learning experiences enhances attainment of instructional objectives by considering the content to be presented and characteristics of the learner.

3.3 Instructional hours are allocated on the basis of instructional objectives, complexity of the content, level of instruction, and resource availability.

3.4 Instructors select instructional media which is current, accurate, and consistent with the instructional objectives.

4. Providers of critical care nursing education select program formats on the basis of instructional objectives and available resources.

RATIONALE:

Selection of the program format provides the framework within which subsequent components of the educational process occur. The appropriateness of the program format ensures that the participants' learning needs and the organization's goals are met within the resource capabilities of the sponsoring agency.

CRITERIA:

4.1 Selection of a program format considers each of the following:
    4.11 The nature of the learning experience
    4.12 The setting most appropriate for the learning experience
    4.13 The size of the learner group
    4.14 The breadth of content to be addressed
    4.15 The level of instruction (beginning, intermediate, or advanced)
    4.16 Application of principles of adult education
    4.17 The amount of time available for preparation and implementation of the program
    4.18 The instructor's experience with the proposed format
    4.19 The availability of resources (human, material, environmental, financial)

5. Providers of critical care nursing education formulate an evaluation strategy during the planning process.

RATIONALE:

Identification of the evaluation strategy is necessary to direct program planning and implementation.

CRITERIA:

5.1 Both program evaluation and evaluation of learning are included in the scope of the evaluation process.

5.2 Providers develop a strategy to evaluate application of learning to critical care nursing practice.

5.3 Providers select and/or design tools for evaluating the program and learning.

5.4 Providers select and validate tools which contain the criteria to be used during the evaluation process.

6. **Providers of critical care nursing education establish criteria for program initiation.**

RATIONALE:

Criteria for program initiation are necessary to decide whether the expenditure of resources can be justified by the anticipated benefits.

CRITERIA:

6.1   Providers delineate prerequisite/entry requirements for each offering within the educational program.
6.2   Providers establish maximum and minimum enrollments for each offering in the educational program.
6.3   Providers select participants based on pre-established criteria.
6.4   Providers establish a time schedule for offerings in the educational program.

Implementation

1. **Providers manage critical care nursing education programs based on the instructional plan.**

RATIONALE:

The effectiveness of an educational offering is dependent upon the selection of appropriate instructional methods. Program goals and objectives guide instructors in selection of appropriate teaching methods.

CRITERIA:

1.1   Program implementation is consistent with the instructional objectives, curriculum, and format selected for the program.
1.2   Program implementation is consistent with the plan for program initiation and the established administrative framework for critical care education programs.

2. **Providers modify how critical care nursing education programs are implemented based on situational variables.**

RATIONALE:

Situational variables such as program timing, availability of facilities and differences among the learners often necessitate alterations in the instructional plan. Modifications are made during the implementation phase to ensure attainment of the program goals and objectives.

CRITERIA:

2.1   Providers use the instructional plan to monitor program operations.
2.2   Providers modify the program based upon discrepancies between planned and actual operations.

3. **Providers of critical care nursing education apply the principles of adult education during program implementation.**

RATIONALE:

Because the learner is an adult, implementation of the program is guided by educational principles that promote adult learning.

CRITERIA:

3.1 Providers afford learners opportunities for active participation in the learning experience.
3.2 Providers incorporate the learners' life and work experiences in instructional activities.
3.3 Providers offer the learners immediate feedback and reinforcement of learning.
3.4 Providers tailor learning experiences toward direct application to critical care nursing practice.

4. **Providers of critical care nursing education create an environment conducive to learning.**

RATIONALE:

A nonjudgmental and nonthreatening environment supports learner participation in the educational process.

CRITERIA:

4.1 Instructors interact with learners in a constructive and supportive manner.
4.2 Instructors establish a climate of openness and mutual respect in their interactions with learners.

Evaluation

1. **Those involved in critical care nursing education programs participate in the evaluation process.**

RATIONALE:

Evaluation is most valid and meaningful when it involves all those directly affected by the results of that evaluation.

CRITERIA:

1.1 Institutional providers evaluate critical care nursing education programs they sponsor.
1.2 Critical care instructors participate in program evaluation.
1.3 Critical care nurses who are directly involved with patient care participate in the evaluation of critical care education programs.
1.4 Critical care nurse managers participate in evaluation of critical care education programs for their staff and other learners.

2. **Providers of critical care nursing education programs evaluate programs in relation to the full scope of critical care nursing practice: the critical care nurse, the critically ill patient, and the environment in which critical care nursing is practiced.**

RATIONALE:

The ultimate aim of critical care nursing education is to ensure the cognitive, affective, and psychomotor components of competency in critical care nursing practice. Since critical care nursing practice encompasses the critical care nurse, patient, and environment, each of these dimensions must be included in any evaluation of a critical care nursing education program.

CRITERIA:

2.1 Providers evaluate program effectiveness in meeting learning needs of the critical care nurse.
2.2 Providers evaluate programs relative to the health needs of the patient populations in critical care areas.
2.3 Providers evaluate programs relative to the realities and constraints of the critical care practice setting.

3. **Providers evaluate critical care nursing education programs relative to predetermined criteria.**

RATIONALE:

Educational programs for critical care nurses must frequently meet concurrent sets of agency, local, regional, and/or national standards, guidelines, and regulations which apply to the learners or to that educational setting.

CRITERIA:

3.1 Providers evaluate critical care education programs relative to their administrative framework.
3.2 Providers evaluate programs relative to the standards of applicable professional accrediting bodies and/or regulatory agencies.
3.3 Providers evaluate programs relative to criteria formulated during program planning.

4. **Those involved in critical care nursing education programs evaluate the effectiveness of each individual offering within the total program.**

RATIONALE:

To determine that an education program has attained its goals, it is necessary to establish that each individual offering within that program has achieved its designated goals.

CRITERIA:

4.1   Providers evaluate the following features of each educational offering:

     4.11   The relevance and priority of instructional objectives for critical care nursing practice

     4.12   The behavioral and measurable attributes of instructional objectives

     4.13   The consistency and correlation between instructional objectives and instructional content

     4.14   The consistency, validity, and correlation between instructional objectives and written and/or clinical evaluation tools used to verify learning acquisition and application

     4.15   The expertise of instructors in facilitating learner attainment of instructional objectives

     4.16   The quality and quantity of classroom, laboratory, and clinical instruction provided

     4.17   The impact of the learning environment in facilitating learning

4.2   Instructors evaluate the following features of each educational offering:

     4.21   The relevance and priority of instructional objectives to critical care nursing practice

     4.22   The consistency and correlation between instructional objectives and the content selected for instruction

     4.23   The correlation and validity between instructional objectives and the written and/or clinical evaluation tools used to verify acquisition and application of learning

     4.24   Their effectiveness as an instructor for that educational offering

     4.25   The effectiveness of the educational setting(s) used for that offering

     4.26   The effectiveness of teaching methods and instructional aids used for that offering

     4.27   The effectiveness of the means employed to evaluate attainment of instructional objectives

     4.28   The effectiveness of the means used to verify application of learning in the practice setting

     4.29   The degree to which teaching-learning principles and principles of adult education were applied

4.3   Learners evaluate the following features of each educational offering:

     4.31   Pertinence and organization of content relative to the instructional objectives

     4.32   The instructional level employed.

     4.33   Time allotted for instruction and integration of learning.

     4.34   Effectiveness of teaching method(s) and instructional aids.

     4.35   Effectiveness of the instructor in facilitating the instructional objectives.

     4.36   Degree to which the instructional setting, environment, and learning climate facilitate learning.

     4.37   Attainment of instructional objectives.

     4.38   Potential for direct application of learning to critical care nursing practice.

4.4 Critical care nurse managers evaluate the following features of each educational offering:

    4.41 The relevance of instructional objectives for role responsibilities of the critical care nurse.

    4.42 Whether the means used for evaluation are valid.

5. Providers of critical care nursing education periodically evaluate the total educational program.

RATIONALE:

Evaluation of a total educational program is necessary to provide information to guide decisions for modification and improvement of subsequent programs. Evaluation of individual educational offerings is incorporated, but is insufficient to afford an overall appraisal of the entire program.

CRITERIA:

5.1 Providers evaluate program effectiveness relative to learners' ability to apply learning in critical care nursing practice.

5.2 Providers evaluate program effectiveness relative to learners' attainment of instructional objectives.

5.3 Providers evaluate program efficiency relative to the resources required to support the program.

5.4 Providers incorporate both formative and summative evaluations of the program.

5.5 Providers periodically revise programs based on the data contained in evaluative records.

——— GLOSSARY

Administrative framework The organizational structure which provides administration and management of the agency or institution.

Clinical nursing instructors Nurses who provide instruction in the clinical setting.

Competency An integration of the cognitive, affective, and psychomotor attributes necessary for performance in a specific role and setting.

Continuing education "Planned organized learning experiences designed to augment the knowledge, skills, and attitudes of registered nurses for the enhancement of nursing practice, education, administration and research, . . . "[1]

Critical care nursing education "Education directed at facilitating application of the knowledge, skills, and attitudes required for competent critical care nursing practice."[2]

Educational offering One segment of a critical care nursing education program. It may be a single experience or activity or a series of experiences or activities.[1]

Educational program Planned, organized learning experiences directed at accomplishing broad educational objectives. A program is comprised of one or more offerings or courses.

Formative evaluation Evaluation performed during the implementation of an educational offering or program.

Instructors Individuals who teach in critical care nursing educational programs.

Outcome standard A statement of quality which defines the educational outcome to be achieved.

Process standard A statement of quality which describes a series of actions, changes, or functions designed to bring about a desired educational outcome.

Program format The arrangement or plan of instruction selected to meet identified educational needs.

Program goals The purposes of the educational program.

Provider An individual or institution responsible for development, implementation, evaluation, and administration of critical care nursing education.

Structure standard A statement of quality which addresses the environment in which critical care nursing education is provided. Structure standards include the administrative framework and human, financial, material, and environmental resources necessary to achieve educational program goals.

Summative evaluation Evaluation performed at the conclusion of an educational offering or program.

REFERENCES

1. American Nurses' Association: Guidelines for Staff Development. Kansas City, 1976, American Nurses' Association, 16-18.
2. Alspach JG: Issues in critical care education. Chicago, 1983, Keynote address, Critical care education: Service perspectives, AACN Leadership Institute.

___Appendix A

CRITICAL CARE NURSING EDUCATION: AN OVERVIEW*

Critical care nursing education is directed at facilitating the application of the knowledge, skills, and attitudes required for competent critical care nursing practice. [1] Since its inception, the American Association of Critical-Care Nurses (AACN) has promoted the advancement of critical care nursing education as a means to provide a high standard of nursing care for the critically ill. Recognizing the diversity of providers and programs, and the inconsistencies in the process of providing critical care nursing education, AACN established the Education Standards Task Force in 1981. The charge of this task force was to develop education standards for critical care nursing.

Characterization of the present state of critical care nursing education was necessary as a frame of reference for developing the education standards. An extensive literature search revealed a scarcity of published research in this area.

This review comprises published reports supplemented by impressions reached by consensus among task force members as experienced nurse educators. A closing segment includes implications for critical care nurse educators, managers, researchers, and practitioners.

Critical care nursing education is provided in three distinct settings: academic, service, and private. For the purpose of the review, each setting is defined. The *academic* setting includes National League for Nursing (NLN)-approved nursing programs in universities, colleges, and hospitals that award a graduate degree, baccalaureate degree, associate degree, or diploma in nursing. Continuing education departments within universities or colleges and academic extension programs are included. Critical care nursing education in this setting is provided as part of basic or graduate nursing education or in the form of continuing education. Continuing education in nursing consists of "planned, organized learning experiences designed to augment the knowledge, skills, and attitudes of registered nurses for the enhancement of nursing practice, education, administration, and research, to the end of improving health care to the public." [2]

---

*Reproduced from *Heart & Lung,* March 1986, vol. 15, no. 2. Used with permission.

Table I ── Components of staff development*

Components	Description	Examples
Orientation	The means by which new staff members are introduced to the philosophy, goals, policies, procedures, role expectations, physical facilities, and special services in a specific work setting; provided during the initial period of employment or role change	Nursing unit or service, hospital, or personnel orientation
In-service education	Learning experiences provided in the work setting for the purpose of assisting staff to perform assigned functions and maintain competency in that particular agency; these experiences are usually narrow in scope and may or may not be formally planned or evaluated	Spontaneous teaching/training situations, question and answer sessions, peer discussions, procedure review, demonstration of new equipment, conferences, unit meetings, and teaching rounds
Continuing education under staff development	Planned, organized learning experiences designed to build on previously acquired knowledge and skills; these activities are directly related to the role expectations of the nurse, and the focus is on knowledge and skills that are not specific to one employment setting or agency; only activities in the continuing education component qualify for the continuing education contact hour	Workshops, formal conferences, seminars, courses, institutes; self-directed learning that is evaluated

*Summarized from Guidelines for staff development. Kansas City, 1978, American Nurses' Association.

The *service* setting includes all health care facilities in which critically ill patients are directly cared for by critical care nurses. While hospitals are the primary source of care for critically ill patients, other facilities such as mobile intensive care units or freestanding emergency clinics are included. In the service setting, critical care nursing education is provided under the category of staff development. Staff development is "a process that includes both formal and informal learning opportunities to assist individuals to perform competently in fulfillment of role expectations with a specific agency."[2] The overlapping components of staff development include orientation, in-service education, and continuing education (Table I).

The *private* setting includes commercial providers or organizations such as proprietary continuing education businesses, vendors, and nursing staff registries that offer critical care programs. Professional associations and societies such as AACN, which offer continuing education for their members, are also part of the private sector. Critical care nursing education in this setting is provided in the form of continuing education.

To characterize critical care nursing education in the three settings, seven features were addressed in the review: (1) the rationale for providing critical care nursing education; (2) the providers (institutional and individual) of critical care nursing education; (3) how critical care nursing education is provided, which includes the components and instructional formats or techniques; (4) the expected outcomes of critical care nursing education; (5) the means by which critical care nursing education is evaluated; (6) the institutional, individual, and professional factors that impinge on critical care nursing education; and (7) existing standards that affect critical care nursing education.

For clarity, competency is defined. *Competency* refers to an intellectual, attitudinal, and/or motor capability derived from a specified role and setting and stated in terms of performance as a broad class or domain of behavior.[3] Competency is the ability to perform a task with desirable outcomes under the varied circumstances of the real world.[4]

——— Rationale for Providing Critical Care Nursing Education

While the ultimate goal of all critical care nursing education programs is to educate nurses for competent practice within the critical care environment, the short-term and intermediate goals differ among the three settings.

Gardam[5] stated that diploma schools of nursing should include critical care nursing education in their curricula to meet society's need for skilled nurses in intensive care units. Geels et al.[6] believed that since most baccalaureate students will be employed in acute care hospitals on graduation, prior experience with patients in the acute stage of illness would be valuable, if not indispensable. In addition, offering an undergraduate critical care course was viewed as a means to bridge the gap between the opposing trends of generalization in collegiate nursing education and specialization in general hospital nursing. Pierce[7] also believed that a baccalaureate, senior-level, critical care experience broadened the scope and depth of general medical-surgical nursing education.

In recognition of a need to prepare nurses to specialize in critical care, Brault and Pflaum[8] developed a graduate-level critical care clinical specialist program. These nurse educators believed that the phenomenal rate of growth of critical care units and the rapid advances in medical science and technology necessitate advanced nursing education. Critical care practitioners and service agencies provide further support for such a program.

One of the primary reasons service providers support continuing education programs is recruitment and retention of qualified staff[9] or to meet the Joint Commission on Accreditation of Hospitals (JCAH) requirements for the training of special care unit nursing staff.[10] No published information was found to substantiate the rationale for providing critical care nursing education in the private setting.

Experience suggests that additional factors motivate providers to offer critical care educational programs. In the service setting, the education of critical care nurses is a high priority. A shortage of adequately trained critical care nurses jeopardizes the ability of the hospital to provide optimal patient care, and most generic nursing programs provide limited, if any, educational experiences in critical care. Consequently, providing orientation programs aimed at ensuring minimal competency in critical care nursing is a necessity.

In-service education is provided to facilitate maintenance of competency, to educate staff on new technology and procedures, to satisfy JCAH requirements, and to offer a professional employee benefit for the staff. Continuing education programs assist a service agency in recruiting and retaining qualified critical care nurses by providing the employee with an opportunity to fulfill educational needs and professional goals.

In the private setting, critical care nursing education is provided in response to perceived or documented learning needs of critical care nurses, service agencies, or the community. Professional associations and societies offer critical care nursing education to assist members to maintain current knowledge or expertise, expand a theoretic base or skill repertoire, maintain specialty certification, meet continuing education requirements for relicensure, or meet other professional learning goals. Likewise, commercial continuing education organizations provide critical care programs that help participants fulfill educational needs, but do so from a proprietary basis. Nursing staff registries that employ critical care nurses frequently provide educational programs to facilitate maintenance of a desired level of competency required by client institutions. Health care product vendors participate in critical care nursing education to facilitate safe and effective use of their products or equipment and to enhance product marketability.

_____ The Providers of Critical Care Nursing Education

Providers of critical care nursing education exist at two distinct levels — institutional and individual. University, college, or school curricula, hospitals, professional health care associations or societies, and commercial companies exemplify institutional providers. Individual providers include academic faculty members, registered nurses, vendor representatives, and other health care professionals (e.g., physicians and respiratory therapists) who participate directly in the education of critical care nurses.

A distinct characterization of these providers could not be derived from the literature. In the academic setting, the accreditation criteria for schools of nursing, as established by the NLN, provide a broad description of the expected qualifications of schools and faculty, but do not specify requirements for critical care nursing education.[11]

In a position statement issued by AACN in 1984 entitled "Integration of Critical Care Nursing Concepts and Clinical Experiences into Professional Nursing Programs," the role responsibilities and qualifications for nursing faculty, professional nursing students, and critical care nurses supervising students were delineated.[12] AACN recommends that nursing faculty and critical care practitioners jointly maintain supervision of students to ensure that practice standards are met and that critical care practitioners retain patient care accountability. Specific requirements for those who supervise nursing students include the following: (1) have a recommended minimum of a baccalaureate degree in nursing for critical care nursing practitioners and a graduate degree appropriate for nursing faculty; (2) demonstrate current clinical expertise in critical care nursing; (3) demonstrate application of knowledge of current critical care nursing literature; and (4) demonstrate application of theoretic knowledge in the clinical supervision of professional nursing students.

Individual providers in the service setting have been characterized as registered nurses who are or have recently been experienced staff nurses in critical care areas and who presently hold a full-time staff position under a title such as critical care instructor, clinical specialist, or staff development instructor. Especially in smaller hospitals, this provider may hold a full-time staff position as a head nurse and be responsible for staff development in addition to management responsibilities.[13] Staff development departments of major medical centers presently constitute the largest group of continuing education providers in nursing.[14]

The preparation of service-based individual providers is also quite variable. Educational levels generally range from diploma preparation in nursing to a master's degree. Typically, the provider has minimal, if any, formal preparation in the staff development educator role and acquires proficiency as an educator through experiential and on-the-job training. Credibility of the critical care educator is rooted in the provider's knowledge and expertise in critical care nursing practice.

The provider's organizational position may be in the critical care service area, the department of staff development, a human resource development department, or the department of nursing education. Staff nurses commonly participate as providers in unit orientation programs in the roles of clinical preceptors.[15] Other agency professionals such as physicians, technicians, and therapists may participate in orientation, in-service, or continuing education offerings for critical care nurses.[1]

In a survey of 28 hospitals, 88% required clinically experienced instructors for their critical care orientation programs. The bachelor of science in nursing degree was accepted as the minimum educational preparation by 38% of the programs and a master's degree by 13%. Staff nurses instructed in 67% of surveyed programs, and non-nursing instructors participated heavily.[16]

No published information could be found that characterized providers in the private sector, but a limited description can be derived from the formal review of critical care continuing education programs submitted to AACN for award of continuing education units. Institutional providers in the category of professional health care associations and societies, e.g., AACN and American Nurses' Association (ANA), represent the second largest provider category of continuing nursing education. Others such as the American College of Chest Physicians and the American Heart Association offer nurses critical care education that is related to that association's respective specialty interests. Individual providers within these organizations may be members, employees, or specialists/practitioners outside of the organization. Faculty qualifications and educational backgrounds vary, but all generally possess some degree of expertise in the content area presented.

Proprietary organizations, a second type of institutional provider in the private setting, include manufacturers of products used in critical care settings, nurse staffing agencies, and continuing education businesses. These providers most commonly employ nurses to plan and implement educational programming. Program faculty may be recruited from internal or external organizational sources, and their qualifications, practice specialties, and backgrounds vary widely. There is currently no agreement on requirements or qualifications of providers in the private setting.

────── How Critical Care Nursing Education is Provided

Subsumed in the process of developing competency in critical care nursing is the acquisition of a specialized body of knowledge and the application of this knowledge to practice. No universally accepted description of the knowledge and practice components could be gleaned from the literature. One attempt to delineate the knowledge basic to safe practice in critical care nursing and a tool to measure that knowledge has been reported. The literature showed that the methods by which these components are acquired can be diverse.

A report published from the 1983 Consensus Development Conference on Critical Care Medicine described the skills essential for intensive care unit (ICU) personnel.[17] Those skills considered to be common to all ICUs included decision making, equipment, procedure, administrative, and teaching and training. Recommendations were that registered nurses should have substantial postgraduate clinical experience before ICU training and that training should include a comprehensive orientation program, followed by on-the-job training with a preceptor.

More detailed outlines of the skills required for competent critical care nursing practice were provided in the form of published curricula for orientation and/or in-service education programs.[13,18-23] The systems approach is the predominant means used to organize the content presented, while nursing process most frequently provided the framework for learning. Common subjects were identified in each curriculum reviewed (Table II). Additional content such as renal dialysis and coagulopathies was considered to be basic content by some authors and advanced by others. Specialized content unique to the type of patients cared for in a given unit (e.g., burn unit) was included in the curriculum in addition to the more generic content.[20,21]

Course content for critical care education programs was determined from various sources (Table III). Documentation on the formats used in critical care education again revealed differences among settings, as well as differences among providers in a given setting. Eight critical care nursing master's programs are identified in *Master's Education in Nursing: Route to Opportunities in Contemporary Nursing 1982-83.*[24] All require a clinical practicum with no formal critical care courses or specific credit hours, and program lengths range from 1 to 2 years. An exception is the three-semester program at California State University at Long Beach, which prepares graduate nurses for competence in practice in cardiovascular, respiratory, neurologic,

Table II ── Basic curriculum content for critical care nursing education[13,18-22]

Cardiopulmonary resuscitation
Arrhythmia interpretation
Hemodynamic monitoring
Mechanical ventilator management
Body fluid monitoring

Table III ── Input sources for course content[18,19,35]

AACN's Core Curriculum for Critical Care Nursing
Other critical care textbooks
Journal articles
Needs surveys
Course evaluations
Student feedback
Faculty feedback
Employer feedback
Supervisor feedback

renal-metabolic, and trauma nursing (a generalist-specialist). A total of 9 credits each in clinical practicum and theory is provided. The latter stress advanced pathophysiology, medical content, and management skills.[8]

At the undergraduate level, Wayne State University School of Nursing offers a critical care elective. Students are coassigned with staff nurses in the clinical area with a student-faculty ratio of 2:1. Clinical and theory components address physiologic and psychological responses to illness, emergency care, assessment skills, self-assessment of learning needs, and identification of professional responsibilities.[6] At the University of North Carolina, a critical care experience, including clinical and theory, was implemented as part of a 14-week health/illness continuum. Students are coassigned to staff nurses in the clinical area with a student/faculty ratio of 8:1.[7] Both programs are offered at the senior level, and credit hours are not specified.

Experience suggests that in the academic setting, critical care education exists almost exclusively at the graduate level and that very limited clinical exposure or theory occurs in generic programs. The general emphasis tends to be on theoretic rather than practice components.

In the service setting, critical care orientation programs vary in length from 1 to 8 weeks. Clinical instruction ranged from 70 to 320 hours and theory instruction from 40 to 125 hours. In the one instance, independent study hours of 200 hours were documented.[16,18,20,22,23] Orientation programs were conducted from two to 12 times per year.[16]

The didactic component of orientation programs tends to be more structured than the clinical and consists of lectures, group discussions, case study reviews, role playing, observations of procedures, and independent study in the form of reading and audiovisual review. Nursing assessment rounds, medical rounds, and skill labora-

Table IV —— Formats for clinical component of orientation programs[15,18,20,33,65-70]

Title	Definition
Preceptorship	One-to-one assignment of an experienced staff nurse with an orientee
Internship	Extended (3 to 12 mo) training period
Buddy system	One experienced staff member responsible for orienting new staff nurse
Coassignment	Pairing of staff member with orientee in dual patient assignment
On-the-job training	Orientee with patient care assignment identifies needs for assistance from a designated resource person

tories are also employed for integrating theory into practice.[13,18,20] Continuing education within the agency consists of a range of learning experiences from lecture presentations to care conferences or workshops.[9,13,25,26]

There are numerous critical care education formats (Table IV). In addition, two relatively independent formats facilitate adult education approaches to critical care orientation. These include self-paced and self-directed learning formats. In a *self-paced* orientation program, the orientee is provided with a preestablished set of expectations for the orientation period. Through the use of readily available resources, the orientee determines how and when various expectations are achieved.[27] A *self-directed* format leaves the identification of learning needs, plans for meeting these needs, and methods of evaluating learning as the prerogative of the orientee with concurrence and/or negotiation with the administrative or educational coordinator.[28-30]

Beyond orientation in the service setting, in-service programs and continuing education are offered. In-service programs usually consist of descriptive presentations or hands-on experiences with new equipment or procedures. Continuing education most frequently involves classroom-based presentations. The degree to which these various formats incorporate principles of teaching, learning, and adult education is extremely variable.

No published information could be found on how critical care education is provided in the private setting. AACN's Continuing Education Approval Program, however, indicates that programs by private providers are most commonly 1- or 2-day lectures or lecture/workshop offerings. Direct clinical instruction is rarely provided. Professional organizations frequently utilize scheduled conference or meeting times to offer additional selected classes or workshops. More recently, private providers have used an increasingly greater number of self-paced learning programs to deliver didactic content. These programs may be in either printed or audiovisual form and may be distributed with a learning evaluation tool that is returned to the provider for processing and for award of continuing education units.

There is much variation on how critical care nursing education is provided. The reason for this variability partly relates to the divergent rationales for providing critical care education in the three educational settings. Factors described under "Factors that Impinge on Critical Care Nursing Education" in this article also influence how critical care education is provided.

——— The Expected Outcomes of Critical Care Nursing Education

Critical care nursing education is expected to prepare a competent critical care nurse and thereby ultimately improve the quality of nursing care to critically ill patients.[17,19] The literature was reviewed for a consensus on the clinical competencies necessary for critical care nursing practice.

In a descriptive study, a panel of experts identified 103 clinical competencies necessary for beginning level practitioners in critical care.[31] Questionnaires to academic nursing faculty and nursing service personnel revealed little agreement between these two groups regarding what clinical competencies were necessary for beginning critical care nurses. The nursing faculty were in closer agreement with the panel of experts than with nursing service personnel.

The expected outcomes of the generic level critical care courses found in the literature were related to student achievement of course objectives.[6,7] At the master's level, specialization in critical care nursing was the expected outcome. According to the ANA,[32] a "... specialist ... is a nurse, who through study and supervised practice (at a graduate level) has become expert in a defined area of knowledge and practice in a selected clinical area."

In the service setting, the expected outcome of critical care orientation programs is that the staff nurse be able to provide safe and competent nursing care to patients on the assigned unit. This level of practice is achieved through mastery of specified skills and acquisition of a specified body of knowledge.[18-21] The expected outcome of critical care in-service education is that the staff nurse maintain and update competency in providing care for patients on the assigned unit.[33] Continued professional development and proficiency as a practitioner in critical care are the expected outcomes of continuing education.[9,34]

Review of critical care programs conducted by private providers indicates that the expected outcomes of these programs largely comprise enabling objectives for cognitive skills. Class-specific instructional objectives generally delineate short-term, learner-centered outcomes that participants are expected to attain by the end of the program (AACN program approval). In theory, it is projected that achievement of course objectives will enable a nurse to maintain current expertise in practice, at least with regard to the knowledge base required for practice.

Experience suggests that the arrival of a critical care nurse at the competent level is largely a subjective determination of evaluators who, for the most part, define competency according to personal or local norms. To date, a complete, empirically derived delineation of essential clinical competencies for critical care nurses has not been elucidated. There are no data correlating competency in critical care nursing practice with positive and measurable patient outcomes. Patient-centered outcomes of critical care nursing education are seldom, if ever, identified. Although the achievement of course objectives as an outcome of some types of critical care education is generally measurable, it is unclear how successful completion of an individual course contributes to overall competency in critical care nursing practice. Provisions for evaluating improvements or changes in clinical practice after continuing education classes are not consistently evidenced.

How Critical Care Nursing Education is Evaluated

Public attention is currently focused on the means of evaluating education and learning. Despite this seemingly high degree of interest, there is a dearth of published information that describes valid and reliable means for evaluating the expected outcomes of critical care nursing education. Some mechanism is generally used to evaluate and document learner attainment of expected outcomes, but the validity and reliability of these mechanisms are rarely scrutinized. Providers in all three educational settings most frequently use written tests to evaluate cognitive learning.[18,19,35] Tests may be objective or subjective and are frequently constructed by individuals who claim some expertise in the content area. The level of questioning in written tests varies, although factual and recall questions seem to predominate. Instructional objectives commonly provide the source of content for cognitive test items.[13,25]

Learning of psychomotor skills is usually evaluated by observation of skills performance by instructors, preceptors, nursing managers, or supervisors.[19,36,37] In all three educational settings, technical skills may be demonstrated in either actual practice situations or in a skills laboratory. Where acquisition of more than an isolated technical competency is desired, evaluative guidelines and a mechanism of documenting skills performance are usually provided by a skills checklist.[18,21,37,38]

Additional methods used to evaluate outcomes of critical care education include care conferences or clinical rounds, care plan audits, peer review, and self-evaluation.[13,18,19] Academic providers may add structured seminars and term papers as means of evaluating cognitive abilities.

The Factors That Impinge on Critical Care Nursing Education

Multiple factors influence the provision of critical care nursing education through effects on programming, providers, and/or participants. For the purpose of this review, these factors are categorized as institutional, professional, and individual.

Institutional factors. In each educational setting, accrediting bodies have a pervasive impact on critical care education programs. The NLN has set forth specific appraisal criteria to serve as standards and guidelines for schools of nursing and faculty in developing and improving educational programs.[24] While these criteria allow flexibility in programming, to some extent they dictate curricular direction through regulation of the consistency between the philosophy, purposes, and conceptual framework of the institution, the school of nursing, and the curriculum. Among these accrediting criteria, specialization in nursing is identified as pertinent only at the level of the second professional degree (master's level). The NLN's position may strongly influence the decision whether to provide generic-level critical care nursing education. ANA also advocates specialization only at the graduate level.[32]

For service agencies, JCAH influences the extent and content of critical care orientation and in-service programs.[39] Health care agencies must meet these educational requirements to maintain accreditation.

Accreditation requirements of continuing education established by state boards of nursing and/or professional nursing associations modify critical care nursing education provided in the private setting. The National Accreditation Board is one accrediting body for continuing education in nursing. Regional accrediting committees, state nurses' associations, and ANA-accredited specialty nursing organizations also have authority to accredit continuing education programs. In those states that have legislated mandatory continuing education for relicensure, state boards of nursing have developed rules and regulations for program sponsors. To receive continuing education unit credit, participants in these states can enroll only in courses offered by state-approved and recognized providers.

Other factors inherent in the service setting impinge on critical care education by affecting the quality of learning experiences encountered by the learner. Patient care priorities, the unavailability of an appropriate patient population for learner experience,[6] inadequate staffing, high staff turnover rates, and/or unavailability of experienced critical care preceptors may color learning experiences. The potential conflict between the philosophy and objectives of a service agency with regard to student education and those of an academic nursing program may also affect student learning in critical care.

Factors such as faculty preparation, student supervision, and the number of clinical contact hours can modify the quantity and quality of critical care education in the academic setting. Even with qualified faculty available, a high student/faculty ratio may reduce the quality of clinical instruction and the degree of clinical supervision possible.[6] An inadequate number of clinical contact hours would make it difficult for students to achieve desired educational outcomes.

The nature of critical care nursing poses additional problems for educating critical care nurses in all three settings. The rapidity of change in this field of practice makes prediction of needed knowledge difficult. Providers must revise and augment programming regularly to keep pace with these changes.[38] In addition, the vastness of the body of critical care knowledge and the expanded scope of critical care units foster specialization.[40] An institution's or provider's material and educational resources to develop and maintain educational programs ultimately determine achievable educational outcomes.[41]

Economic factors have a pervasive influence over the provision of critical care education in all settings. Although financial resources may not exclusively determine whether a critical care program is provided, fiscal realities significantly influence the number and nature of programs provided. Economics force a provider to rank needs and choose how to allocate resources for educational programming.

Service agencies, subjected to the prospective reimbursement system, as well as other cost-containment programs, may become less able to offer educational benefits to their employees. Nurses may be required to finance their own education and attend programs on their off-duty time. These factors may reduce a nurse's ability and motivation to pursue additional education external to the programs provided within the agency.

The decreased ability of service agencies to subsidize employees' attendance at educational programs in turn affects private and academic providers. As the economy becomes tighter, profits are reduced to make programs more affordable to participants. Thus, the programs offered will tend to be proven, well-attended programs rather than newer or more innovative ones that may carry a greater risk of financial failure. The room rates an institution may charge to generate revenue are regulated in some states. This could adversely affect the number of critical care programs provided by that agency and diminish the funds available for subsidizing continuing education for nursing staff.

The number, type, and diversity of patients served by a given health care facility, as well as the scientific and technologic sophistication in the agency, influence the content and extent of critical care education required for staff.[42] Policies, procedures, and certification requirements established in a nursing services department, changes in nursing practice,[43] and quality assurance activities operating in a service agency[44] determine to some extent staff-training requirements for critical care practice.

Professional factors. Multiple professional factors have ramifications for critical care nursing education in all three educational settings. Academic and service providers appear to be more directly affected by these factors than are private providers.

In the academic setting, controversy surrounding nursing education at the generic level frustrates efforts at defining specialty nursing education. A differentiation of the levels of nursing practice among graduates of associate degree, diploma, and baccalaureate nursing programs, as well as the delineation of competencies nursing graduates should uniformly possess, have not materialized.[40,45,46] Without these standards as points of reference, it is unlikely that generic-level critical care nursing education could be clearly distinguished.

Significant disagreement exists between nursing educators and nursing service employers regarding what core competencies are necessary for beginning critical care nursing practice.[31] Such conflicts tend to influence the content and extent of critical care programs provided in each setting, particularly with respect to the clinical component.

Also operative in the service settings are factors such as nurse practice acts that dictate the legal scope of nursing practice within a given state and that state's requirements for licensure and relicensure of professional nurses.[47,48] Only a minority of states presently require mandatory continuing education for relicensure.[49,50]

Political, legal, and governmental factors impinge on the nursing profession in the work setting through influence over legislation,[51] training funds for health care workers, health insurance reimbursements, and the outcomes of litigation related to practicing nurses.[52]

Practice within critical care areas is influenced by modifications of nurse-physician roles and functions. Nurses have gradually acquired numerous role responsibilities previously within the realm of medical practice.[13] In turn, nurses delegate segments of their task responsibilities to growing numbers of paraprofessionals and ancillary health care workers.

Other professional issues affecting critical care education include contemporary systems of health care delivery, codes of ethics, and standards of practice, as well as findings of nursing research. Certification programs offered for general or specialty nursing practitioners attempt to validate attainment of a specific level of nursing practice and/or the acquisition of a defined body of knowledge; the requirements of these certification programs clearly dictate educational direction.

Individual factors. Individual factors affecting critical care nursing education alter the learner's motivation toward critical care education. Documentation of these factors in relation to service-based and service-supported staff development offerings is available.[53-55] Family, financial, administrative, and peer support systems[56-58] and geographic location may present actual or perceived obstacles to attendance at educational programs. Professional accountability and growth, career and status progression,[59] financial and work-time incentives,[60,61] and the nurse's full- or part-time employment status further influence the critical care nurse's participation in staff development programs.

Although not described in the literature, some of these same individual factors are believed to influence participation in critical care programs in the private setting and in academic-based continuing education programs. In states where mandatory continuing education is legislated and financial assistance for education from employers is limited, critical care nurses may be more apt to choose educational programs based on their proximity to home or work and their cost rather than according to legitimate educational needs. Although participation in continuing education is significantly reduced when it is not required either by law, employers, or certification status, critical care nurses may seek only those programs they consider to be relevant to their practice or professional advancement.

—— Existing Sets of Standards Affecting Critical Care Nursing Education

Professional standards offer quality statements relative to critical care education in the service and academic settings. No standards were located with implications exclusively for critical care education in the private setting, although private providers frequently follow the guidelines for accreditation of continuing education programs set forth by State Boards of Nursing and professional nursing associations.

Criteria for the appraisal of academic nursing programs were the only standards found relevant to this setting. *NLN Criteria for the Appraisal of Baccalaureate and Higher Degree Programs in Nursing*[11] broadly addresses the organization and administration, students, faculty, curriculum, and resources, facilities, and services of schools granting baccalaureate and graduate degrees in nursing. Similar criteria exist for diploma programs[62] and programs leading to an associate degree.[63] Specialty nursing education is not specifically addressed in these criteria, yet several criteria have implications for critical care nursing education. Specific criteria state that faculty have graduate preparation and experience appropriate to areas of responsibility and that they continue to improve their expertise.

In the service setting, the professional standards relevant to critical care education include AACN's *Standards for Nursing Care of the Critically Ill,*[64] ANA's

Standards for Continuing Education in Nursing,[34] ANA's *Guidelines for Staff Develop-ment,*[2] and JCAH accreditation criteria.[10] AACN practice standards require that nurses demonstrate that they possess the knowledge base, psychomotor skills, and ability to integrate these into clinical practice before assuming independent responsibility for patient care. Other areas addressed in specific standards include the individual's responsibility for maintaining competency and the specific content of critical care orientation programs.

_____ Summary and Implications

As an initial step in developing education standards for critical care nursing and providing a framework for the implementation and evaluation of the impact of these standards, the literature was reviewed to characterize critical care nursing education as it currently exists. Seven pertinent features of critical care nursing education were examined in relation to the three settings in which critical care education is provided.

The literature reveals much variability and inconsistency in the process and structure of critical care nursing education in the academic, service, and private settings. Universal standards and guidelines are not available. Although the rationale for providing critical care nursing education is to prepare competent critical care practitioners, specific short-term and intermediate goals vary among the three settings because of the nature of the organization.

Institutional and individual providers of critical care education possess varied credentials and educational preparation. There is no consensus on what qualifications or educational competencies are essential for providers of critical care education to effect desired educational outcomes. The methods and formats employed by provid-ers of critical care education to facilitate learning of the clinical and didactic compo-nents of critical care also vary considerably. Opinions differ regarding what constitutes core knowledge and skills, thus affecting the course content and format of programs. Furthermore, the degree to which teaching and adult learning principles are incor-porated into critical care educational methods could not be determined.

Although the expected outcomes of critical care nursing education are to prepare a competent critical care nurse and ultimately to improve the quality of nursing care of the patient, no data could be found correlating competency in practice with positive patient outcomes. The influence of continuing education on critical care nursing practice is largely unknown and inferred.

Descriptions of various methods used to evaluate critical care nursing educa-tion can be found in the existing literature, but the reliability and validity of these methods have not been substantiated. Written tests are most commonly used to evalu-ate cognitive learning, while clinical skills are commonly evaluated by observation. In many instances, evaluation of learning is confused with evaluation of the program, learning environment, or learner satisfaction.

The institutional, professional, and individual factors that affect the provision of critical care nursing education in the three settings were reviewed in the literature.

The full impact of these factors on critical care educational programming, providers, and participants could not be discerned.

Professional standards that relate to critical care education were examined. In the service and academic settings, several standards, although limited in scope, offer statements of quality encompassing structure, process, and outcome criteria relevant to critical care nursing education. No standards specifically tailored for critical care education in the private sector were found, but standards exist that apply to all three settings for continuing education in nursing.

In the absence of established standards, critical care educators, staff, managers, health care administrators, academic institutions, and the general public have no assurance that valid educational processes and structures exist in the field of critical care nursing education. Standards for critical care nursing education would provide a means to ensure that a valid educational process is used and that nursing care of critically ill patients would ultimately be enhanced.

———— Areas for Research in Critical Care Nursing Education

From the overall scarcity of published data on the topic, it is evident that much research in the area of critical care nursing education is warranted. To stimulate further thought and facilitate an interchange of ideas among critical care nurses, the following list of broad researchable questions is offered.

1. What minimal competencies (cognitive, psychomotor, or affective) are necessary to ensure safe and effective clinical practice for critical care nurses? What competencies define the bounds of "intermediate" or "advanced" practice of critical care nursing? What competencies define specialization in critical care nursing?

2. To what degree and in what form are the various educational methods, formats, and/or vehicles effective in facilitating attainment of desired critical care competencies?

3. What evaluative methods and/or instruments will provide valid and reliable measures of competency in critical care nursing?

4. What structural components are required to effect a valid critical care educational process? More specifically, what is optimal with regard to the: (a) qualifications, requirements, and responsibilities of institutional and individual providers of critical care education in each educational setting; (b) educational resources (material, financial, and human) required for critical care education; (c) environmental and instructional supports; (d) staffing and instructor/learner ratios; and (e) organizational and managerial support for critical care education?

5. What patient outcomes correlate positively with competency in critical care nursing?

6. Which methods of assessment will ensure valid, accurate, and reliable identification of learning needs of critical care nurses?

7. To what extent and in what manner do various institutional, professional, and individual factors influence the provision of critical care nursing education?

REFERENCES

1. Alspach JG: Issues in critical care education. Keynote address. Presented at AACN Leadership Institute, Chicago, 1983.
2. Guidelines for staff development. Kansas City, 1978, American Nurses' Association.
3. Cyrs TE, Dobbert DJ: A competency-based curriculum—what is it? Minneapolis, 1976, College of Pharmacy, University of Minnesota.
4. Benner P: Issues in competency-based testing. Nurs Outlook 30:303, 1982.
5. Gardam J: Observations on intensive care units. Supervisor Nurse 18:24, 1972.
6. Geels WJ, Brand LM, Passos JY: The ICU and collegiate nursing education. J Nurs Educ 13:15, 1974.
7. Pierce SF: Clinical experience in the intensive care unit. Nurs Outlook 25:650, 1977.
8. Brault GL, Pflaum S: Planning and development of a master's degree program in critical care. Heart Lung 8:933, 1979.
9. Tobin HM, Wise PSY, Hull PK: The process of staff development. Ed. 2. St. Louis, 1979, The C.V. Mosby Co.
10. Joint Commission on Hospital Accreditation. Accreditation manual for hospitals. Chicago, 1984.
11. Criteria for the appraisal of baccalaureate and higher degree programs in nursing. Publication No. 15-1251. New York, 1977, National League for Nursing.
12. Position statement: Integration of critical care nursing concepts and clinical experiences into entry level professional nursing programs. Newport Beach, Calif., 1983, American Association of Critical-Care Nurses.
13. Alspach JG: The educational process in critical care nursing. St. Louis, 1982, The C.V. Mosby Co.
14. Strauss MB, Abruzzese RS, Yoder PS, et al: The scope of continuing nursing education as a field of practice. J Contin Educ Nurs 13:13, 1982.
15. Moyer MG, Mann JK: A preceptorship program of orientation within the critical care unit. Heart Lung 8:530, 1979.
16. Gottschall MA, Bennetta P, Klee S, et al: Critical care orientation programs. Nurs Mgt 14:32, 1983.
17. Critical care medicine—consensus conference. JAMA 250:798, 1983.
18. Holloway N: Nursing the critically ill adult. Menlo Park, Calif., 1979, Addison-Wesley Publishing Co.
19. Zschoche DA: Critical care education. In Mosby's comprehensive review of critical care. St. Louis, 1976, The C.V. Mosby Co.
20. Rieman MD: Educational approaches to burn nursing orientation, J Burn Care Rehabil 4:30, 1983.
21. Huang S, Dasher L, Varner C: Performance appraisal for CCU nurses. Nurs Mgr 12:50, 1981.
22. Torrez MR: Educational needs of the coronary care nurse. Heart Lung 1:254, 1972.
23. LaFontan L: An approach to ICU nurse education in a small, rural, community hospital. J Cont Educ Nurs 2:32, 1971.
24. Master's education in nursing: route to opportunities in contemporary nursing 1982-83. Publication No. 15-1312. New York, 1982, National League for Nursing.
25. Clark CC: The nurse as continuing educator. New York, 1979, Springer Verlag.
26. Popiel ES: Nursing and the process of continuing education. St. Louis, 1977, The C.V. Mosby Co.
27. Hansell HN, Foster SB: Critical care nursing orientation: a comparison of teaching methods. Heart Lung 9:1066, 1980.
28. Cooper SS: Self-directed learning in nursing. Wakefield, Mass., 1980, Nursing Resources.

29. Puntillo K, Duncan J: An alternative learning experience for intensive care unit nurses. J Cont Educ Nurs 11:44, 1980.
30. Harrell JRS: Orienting the experienced critical care nurse. Supervisor Nurse 11:32, 1980.
31. Canfield A: Clinical competencies for critical care nurses. West J Nurs Res 3:272, 1981.
32. American Nurses' Association Congress for Nursing Practice: Nursing: a social policy statement. Kansas City, 1980, American Nurses' Association.
33. Alspach JG: Improving critical care orientation. Seminar materials, Resource Applications. Baltimore, 1983.
34. Standards for continuing education in nursing. Kansas City, 1984, American Nurses' Association.
35. Toth JC, Ritchey KA: New from nursing research: the basic knowledge assessment tool (BKAT) for critical care nursing. Heart Lung 13:272, 1984.
36. Voorman D: President's message — acute pedagogical crisis . . . critical care intervention. Heart Lung 5:191, 1976.
37. McCaffrey C: Performance checklists. Nurse Educator 3:11, 1978.
38. Freeman A, McMaster D, Hamilton L: Staff development program for critical care nurses. Crit Care Nurse 2:86, 1983.
39. Clough JA: Developing and implementing orientation to a critical care unit. Focus on AACN 9:24, 1982.
40. Wang R, Watson J: The professional nurse: roles, competencies and characteristics. Supervisor Nurse 8:69, 1977.
41. Harris H: The coming recession: how it will affect training and what you can do to survive. Training/Hrd 16:32, 1979.
42. Benner P: From novice to expert. Am J Nurs 82:402, 1982.
43. Benner P: Uncovering the knowledge embedded in clinical practice. Image 15:36, 1983.
44. Smeltzer CH, Feltman B, Rajki K: Nursing quality assurance: a process, not a tool. J Nurs Adm 13:5, 1983.
45. Nelson L: Competence of nursing graduates in technical, communicative, and administrative skills. Nurs Res 27:121, 1978.
46. McLane A: Core competencies of masters-prepared nurses. Nurs Res 27:48, 1978.
47. Kelly LY: Licensure laws in transition. Nurs Outlook 30:375, 1982.
48. Weisfeld N, Falk D: Chasing elusive competence. Hospitals 57:61, 1983.
49. Puetz BE: Who stays away from continuing education? And why? Focus Contin Educ 3:22, 1982.
50. CE now required for relicensure in 16 states. Am J Nurs 82:1668, 1982.
51. Mandatory continuing education: The legislative state of the art. Kansas City, 1978, American Nurses' Association.
52. American Nurses' Association: NLN praises Institute of Medicine report. Hospitals 57:49, 1983.
53. Edelstein RRG, Bunnell M: Determinants of continuing nursing education. J Contin Educ Nurs 9:19, 1978.
54. O'Connor AB: The continuing nurse learner: who and why? Nurse Educator 5:24, 1980.
55. Schoen DC: Lifelong learning: how some participants see it. J Contin Educ Nurs 10:3, 1979.
56. Erickson H: Coping with new systems. J Nurs Educ 22:132, 1983.
57. Turnbull E: Rewards in nursing: the case of nurse preceptors. J Nurs Adm 13:10, 1983.
58. Pinter K: Support systems for health professions students. J Nurs Educ 22:232, 1983.
59. Sovie MD: Fostering professional nursing careers in hospitals: the role of staff development, part 2. J Nurs Adm 13:30, 1983.
60. Lesher DC, Bomberger AS: The roving inservice — an innovative approach to learning J Contin Educ Nurs 14:19, 1983.

61. Carlson S: Twenty-four hour staff education. J Nurs Adm 13:2, 1983.
62. Criteria for the evaluation of diploma programs in nursing. Publication No. 16-1370. New York, 1982, National League for Nursing.
63. Criteria for the evaluation of educational programs in nursing leading to an associate degree. Publication No. 23-1258. New York, 1982. National League for Nursing.
64. Thierer J, Perhus S, McCracken ML, Reynolds MA, Holmes AM, Turton B, Berkowitz DS, Disch JM, editors: Standards for Nursing Care of the Critically Ill. American Association of Critical-Care Nurses. Reston, Va., 1981, Reston Publishing Co.
65. Zwolski K: Preceptors for critical care areas. Focus on AACN 9:7, 1982.
66. May L: Clinical preceptors for new nurses. Am J Nurs 80:1824, 1980.
67. Alspach J: A critical care nursing internship program. Supervisor Nurse 9:31, 1978.
68. Holmes AM, Perez IL, Duffy CM: Critical care nursing internship: a solution to the acute shortage. Crit Care Med 9:114, 1981.
69. Bitgood G: Critical care nurse-intern program. Supervisor Nurse 7:42, 1976.
70. delBueno DJ, Quaife MC: Special orientation units pay off. Am J Nurs 76:1629, 1976.

—Appendix B

**A NATIONAL SURVEY OF CRITICAL CARE
NURSING EDUCATION: SURVEY
QUESTIONNAIRE**

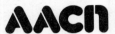 **AMERICAN ASSOCIATION OF CRITICAL-CARE NURSES**

Education Standards Task Force

Chairperson
JoAnn Grif Alspach, RN, MSN, CCRN

Board Liaison
Wanda Roberts, RN, MN, CCRN

Members
Judith Bell, RN, EdD
Mary Canobbio, RN, MN
Susan B. Christoph, RN, DNSc, CCRN
Clareen Wiencek, RN, MSN, CCRN

Staff Liaison
Lane Turzan, RN, MN

Dear Colleague:

On behalf of AACN and the Education Standards Task Force, I would like to thank you for agreeing to participate in the first national survey of critical care nursing education.

Your assistance with this project is vitally important. The information obtained from this study will be published by AACN for the benefit of critical care nurses around the world. Findings will also be used as baseline data for evaluating the education standards for critical care nursing. All survey data will be kept confidential and will be processed in an anonymous fashion.

The study instrument is enclosed. Instructions for completing this form appear on the study itself. In order to incorporate your input into the findings, we will need to receive your responses by 17 days from the mailing date. Please return the study to ASI in the postage-paid envelope provided.

Thank you in advance for your assistance in this project.

Sincerely,

Grif Alspach, RN, MSN, CCRN
Chairperson, Education Standards Task Force

 National Office: One Civic Plaza, Suite 330, Newport Beach, CA 92660 ☐ (714) 644-9310

Part I: Background Information Section

This information is confidential and will be used for data analysis purposes only. For example, we will need to determine how many respondents were from a particular region of the country in order to judge whether the sample is representative. Please indicate your choice(s) by blackening the appropriate circles.

1. Sex:

   ① Male
   ② Female

2. Age:

   ① 20-29
   ② 30-39
   ③ 40-49
   ④ 50+

3. Nursing Education (indicate the highest level completed):

   Nursing   Other
   ① AD   ⑥ Bachelor's degree in _____
   ② Diploma   ⑦ Master's degree in _____
   ③ Bachelor's   ⑧ Doctoral degree in _____
   ④ Master's
   ⑤ Doctorate

4. Primary Area of Practice:

   ① Administration: Director of Critical Care Nursing
   ②   Head Nurse
   ③   Supervisor
   ④ Educational: Director of Critical Care Education
   ⑤   Critical Care Instructor
   ⑥ Staff Nurse
   ⑦ Clinical Nurse Specialist
   ⑧ Private Practice: Business
   ⑨   Continuing Nursing Education Provider
   ⑩ Professional Nursing Association

5. Employment:

   ① Part-time
   ② Full-time

6. Primary Employment Setting:

 ① Nonprofit
 ② For-profit

7. Primary Practice Setting:

 ① Community Hospital
 ② University Teaching Hospital
 ③ Military or Federal Hospital

   If hospital-based, indicate the number of beds in work setting:
   ⓐ fewer than 50
   ⓑ 50-99
   ⓒ 100-199
   ⓓ 200-299
   ⓔ 300-399
   ⓕ 400+
   GO TO QUESTION 8.

 ④ Academic Institution

   If academic-based, indicate the total number of students in your institution:
   ⓐ fewer than 5,000
   ⓑ 5,000-7,999
   ⓒ 8,000-10,999
   ⓓ 11,000-13,999
   ⓔ 14,000-16,999
   ⓕ 17,000-19,999
   ⓖ 20,000+
   GO TO QUESTION 8.

 ⑤ Business

   If business-based, indicate the number of employees:
   ⓐ self employed/solo practice
   ⓑ 2-9
   ⓒ 10-20
   ⓓ 21+
   GO TO QUESTION 8.

 ⑥ Association

   If association-based, indicate the number of employees:
   ⓐ fewer than 3
   ⓑ 3-29
   ⓒ 30-49
   ⓓ 50-99
   ⓔ 100+
   GO TO NEXT QUESTION.

8. In which geographic region do you practice?
   ① Region 1 (CT, MA, ME, NH, RI, VT)
   ② Region 2 (PA, NJ, NY)
   ③ Region 3 (DE, DC, FL, GA, MD, NC, SC, VA, WV)
   ④ Region 4 (IL, IN, MI, OH, WI)
   ⑤ Region 5 (AL, KY, MS, TN)
   ⑥ Region 6 (IA, KS, MN, MO, NE, ND, SD)
   ⑦ Region 7 (AR, LA, OK, TX)
   ⑧ Region 8 (AZ, CO, ID, MT, NM, NV, UT, WY)
   ⑨ Region 9 (AK, CA, HI, OR, WA)

9. Which of the following locations best describes your practice area?
   ① Rural
   ② Suburban
   ③ Urban

10. Number of years of experience in critical care education:
    ① fewer than 2
    ② 2-3
    ③ 4-5
    ④ 6-10
    ⑤ 11-15
    ⑥ 16-20
    ⑦ 20+

11. Number of years of experience in critical care nursing:
    ① fewer than 2
    ② 2-3
    ③ 4-5
    ④ 6-10
    ⑤ 11-15
    ⑥ 16-20
    ⑦ 20+

12. Which of the following professional nursing certifications do you hold (check all that apply)?
    ① CRNA
    ② CCRN
    ③ CEN
    ④ CNRN
    ⑤ CVNS
    ⑥ CNOR
    ⑦ RNC
    ⑧ RNCS

Part II: Organizational Structure

Check all of the following elements that currently exist in your organization. Then indicate how useful each element is to critical care nursing education.

Usefulness
0 does not apply
1 not useful
2 moderately useful
3 quite useful
4 extremely useful

	Which apply? (Check those which exist in your organization)	Usefulness (Rate all elements)
1. Written philosophy	☐	☐
2. Written organizational chart	☐	☐
3. Written policies and procedures	☐	☐
4. Program review by accrediting bodies	☐	☐
5. Internal program review	☐	☐
6. Follow-up on educational quality assurance outcomes	☐	☐
7. Periodic performance appraisals for those providing critical care nursing	☐	☐
8. Written mechanism for budget development	☐	☐
9. Position descriptions for all involved in critical care nursing education	☐	☐
10. Documentation of the outcomes of the needs assessment	☐	☐
11. Documentation of program planning	☐	☐
12. Documentation of program budget	☐	☐
13. Documentation of actual revenue and expenses	☐	☐
14. Documentation of attendance	☐	☐
15. Documentation of program evaluation	☐	☐
16. Documentation of qualifications of providers	☐	☐

Human Resources

17. How many critical care instructors are in your setting? .... **Number** ☐

For each instructor, indicate his/her educational background:

Instructor (No.)	A Highest Degree 1-Diploma 2-Associate 3-Bachelor's 4-Master's 5-Doctorate	B # hours of orientation to position as instructor	C Average # hours of continuing education per year	D # of academic courses in education	E # courses in clinical specialty
18. #1					
19. #2					
20. #3					
21. #4					
22. #5					
23. #6					
24. #7					
25. #8					
26. #9					
27. #10					
28. #11					
29. #12					
30. #13					
31. #14					
32. #15					

Indicate the number of **other** health care professionals who provide critical care education in your organization:

Number

33. Non-critical-care nurses .... ☐

34. Physicians .... ☐

35. Other (please list occupation(s)): ————————————————— .... ☐

For critical care **clinical** nursing instructors:

36. What percent of instructors meet the nursing practice standards of the critical care unit in their area of teaching assignment? .... ☐ %

37. What percent of instructors demonstrate competence in the application of nursing and scientific concepts and principles to care of the critically ill patient? .... ☐ %

38. Are the existing selection criteria for critical care nursing instructors consistent with program goals?

                          1=Not very much   ☐
                          2=Moderately
                          3=Quite
                          4=Extremely

    Indicate the average ratio of instructors:learners for: Instructors : Learners

39. Classroom instructors to learners . . . .   ☐ : ☐

40. Clinical instructors to learners . . . .   ☐ : ☐

41. To what degree does the clinical instructor:learner ratio ensure patient safety?

                          1=Not very much   ☐
                          2=Moderately
                          3=Quite
                          4=Extremely

Indicate the number and sufficiency of support personnel available to facilitate attainment of program goals:

                          1=Insufficient
                          2=Somewhat sufficient
                          3=Moderately sufficient
                          4=Completely sufficient

                                                                    Number   Sufficiency

42. Secretarial staff . . . .   ☐   ☐

43. Audiovisual staff . . . .   ☐   ☐

44. Maintenance staff . . . .   ☐   ☐

45. Biomedical engineering staff . . . .   ☐   ☐

46. Other (please list occupation(s)): _____ . . . . . .   ☐   ☐

For each of the following statements, indicate both the frequency with which each element occurs in your setting and its usefulness to critical care nursing education activities:

Frequency	Usefulness
0=does not apply	0=does not apply
1=never	1=not useful
2=seldom	2=moderately useful
3=sometimes	3=quite useful
4=frequently	4=extremely useful
5=always	

Financial Resources

Freq. Use.

47. A mechanism is used for comparison and analysis between program budget and actual program revenues and expenses .... ☐ ☐

48. A mechanism is used to relate outcomes of financial analysis to attainment of program goals .... ☐ ☐

49. Financial resources are adequate to meet program goals .... ☐ ☐

Please indicate the primary and, if appropriate, secondary source of financial support as it applies to your setting:

Primary   Secondary
(check one)   (check one)

50. If academic setting:

Participant-supported .... ☐ ☐

Employer-supported (nongovernment) .... ☐ ☐

Government .... ☐ ☐

51. If private continuing education setting:

Participant-supported .... ☐ ☐

Employer-supported (nongovernment) .... ☐ ☐

Government .... ☐ ☐

52. If hospital-based setting:

Participant-supported .... ☐ ☐

Employer-supported (nongovernment) .... ☐ ☐

Government .... ☐ ☐

Frequency
0=does not apply
1=never
2=seldom
3=sometimes
4=frequently
5=always

Usefulness
0=does not apply
1=not useful
2=moderately useful
3=quite useful
4=extremely useful

Material Resources

Freq. Use.

53. Material resources used in critical care nursing education programs are consistent with the instructional objectives ....

54. Instructional aids are accurate and current ....

55. Up-to-date reference materials are available to providers ....

56. Up-to-date reference materials are available to participants ....

57. Sufficient reference materials are available to providers ....

58. Sufficient reference materials are available to participants ....

Environmental Resources

59. Physical facilities are conducive to attainment of program goals and instructional objectives ....

60. Physical facilities allow for flexibility in teaching methods, learning styles, and program scheduling ....

61. Physical facilities are accessible to providers ....

62. Physical facilities are accessible to participants ....

64. Storage space is available for material resources and educational records ......

65. Storage space is accessible for material resources and educational records ....

66. Clinical experiences are available to meet the instructional objectives related to nursing practice ....

Assessment of Learning Needs

67. Learners have primary responsibility for the identification of their own learning needs ....

68. Critical care supervisors assist learners in identifying individual and collective learning needs ....

69. Critical care instructors assist learners in identifying individual and collective learning needs ....

70. Providers of critical care education programs facilitate the assessment of learning needs ....

71. Individuals who participate in identifying learning needs take responsibility for communicating their findings to the providers of critical care nursing education ....

72. Providers assess the validity and reliability of methods used for collection of assessment data prior to data analysis ....

73. Providers analyze trends in assessment information ....

Frequency
0 does not apply
1 never
2 seldom
3 sometimes
4 frequently
5 always

Usefulness
0 does not apply
1 not useful
2 moderately useful
3 quite useful
4 extremely useful

Freq. Use.

74. Providers analyze the credibility of assessment information sources .... ☐ ☐

75. Prior to program planning, providers collaborate with critical care practitioners, supervisors, administrators and instructors to validate conclusions drawn during the assessment process .... ☐ ☐

76. Providers establish priorities among learning needs relative to the philosophy and goals of the program and available resources .... ☐ ☐

77. Prior to participation in a critical care education program, the learner assesses the congruence between his/her own learning needs and the goals and objectives of the educational program .... ☐ ☐

78. Before repeating a critical care education program, providers verify the nature and priority of learning needs .... ☐ ☐

Indicate both the frequency with which the following data-gathering devices are used and their usefulness in determining learning needs and goals. Use the rating scales presented below:

Frequency
0 does not apply
1 never
2 seldom
3 sometimes
4 frequently
5 always

Usefulness
0 does not apply
1 not useful
2 moderately useful
3 quite useful
4 extremely useful

Freq. Use.

79. Surveys, reports, questionnaires, marketing response .... ☐ ☐

80. Direct observations of critical care practice .... ☐ ☐

81. Results of quality assurance activities .... ☐ ☐

82. Established standards of nursing care....................................... ☐ ☐

83. Current professional literature.. ☐ ☐

84. Position descriptions and performance appraisals .... ☐ ☐

85. Administrative policies, procedures and directives .... ☐ ☐

86. Prior program evaluations .... ☐ ☐

87. Recommendations from consumers of health services .... ☐ ☐

Resources to Achieve Program Goals

Indicate the frequency with which the following items are analyzed to determine the compatibility between resources and program goals. Use the rating scale presented below:

Frequency
1 never
2 seldom
3 sometimes
4 frequently
5 always

Freq.

88. Organizational structure . . . . □

89. Human resources . . . . □

90. Financial services . . . . □

91. Environmental resources . . . . □

92. Material resources . . . . □

Program Goals and Objectives

Frequency	Usefulness
0 does not apply	0 does not apply
1 never	1 not useful
2 seldom	2 moderately useful
3 sometimes	3 quite useful
4 frequently	4 extremely useful
5 always	

Freq.   Use.

93. Program goals reflect the established priority of learning needs identified during the assessment process . . . . □ □

94. Instructional objectives are consistent with and further define the program goals . . . . □ □

95. Instructional objectives identify the cognitive, psychomotor, and/or affective behavior the learner will demonstrate following program participation . . . . □ □

96. Instructional objectives include application of knowledge and/or skills . . . . □ □

97. Instructional objectives include clearly stated and measurable performance expectations of learners . . . . □ □

98. Content of the curriculum is selected and leveled to facilitate learner attainment of the instructional objectives . . . . □ □

99. The sequencing of learning experiences considers the content to be presented and characteristics of the learner (educational and experiential background) . . . . □ □

100. Instructional hours are allocated on the basis of instructional objectives, complexity of the content, level of instruction, and resource availability . . . . □ □

Frequency
0 does not apply
1 never
2 seldom
3 sometimes
4 frequently
5 always

Usefulness
0 does not apply
1 not useful
2 moderately useful
3 quite useful
4 extremely useful

Freq. Use.

101. Providers select instructional media that are current, accurate, and consistent with the instructional objectives . . . . ☐ ☐

Program Formats

Selection of a program format considers each of the following elements:

102. Size of the learner group . . . . ☐ ☐

103. Breadth of content to be addressed . . . . ☐ ☐

104. Level of instruction (beginning, intermediate, or advanced) . . . . ☐ ☐

105. Application of principles of adult education . . . . ☐ ☐

106. Amount of time available for preparation and implementation of the program . . . . ☐ ☐

107. Providers' experience with the formats considered . . . . ☐ ☐

108. Availability of resources (human, material, environmental, financial) . . . . ☐ ☐

Evaluation Strategy

109. Both program evaluation and evaluation of learning are included in the evaluation process . . . . ☐ ☐

110. Providers develop a strategy to evaluate application of learning to critical care nursing practice . . . . ☐ ☐

111. Providers select and/or design tools for evaluating the program and learning . . . . ☐ ☐

112. Providers select and validate tools which contain the criteria to be used during the evaluation process . . . . ☐ ☐

Program Implementation

113. Providers establish maximum and minimum enrollments for each offering in the educational program . . . . ☐ ☐

114. Providers delineate prerequisite/entry requirements for each offering within the educational program . . . . ☐ ☐

115. Providers select participants based on pre-established criteria . . . . ☐ ☐

116. Providers establish a time schedule of offerings in the educational program . . . ☐ ☐

117. Program implementation is consistent with the instructional objectives, curriculum and format selected for the program . . . . ☐ ☐

118. Program implementation is consistent with the plan for program initiation and the established administrative framework for critical care educational programs . . . . ☐ ☐

Frequency
0=does not apply
1=never
2=seldom
3=sometimes
4=frequently
5=always

Usefulness
0=does not apply
1=not useful
2=moderately useful
3=quite useful
4=extremely useful

119. Providers use instructional and management plans to monitor program operations .... ☐ ☐

120. Providers modify the program based upon discrepancies between planned and actual implementation .... ☐ ☐

121. Providers afford learners opportunities for active participation in the learning experience .... ☐ ☐

122. Providers incorporate the learners' life and work experience in instructional activities .... ☐ ☐

123. Providers offer learners immediate feedback and reinforcement of learning ... ☐ ☐

124. Providers tailor learning experiences toward direct application of critical care nursing practice .... ☐ ☐

125. Instructors interact with learners in a constructive and supportive manner..... ☐ ☐

126. Instructors establish a climate of openness and mutual respect in their interactions with learners .... ☐ ☐

Number of critical care courses offered:

If hospital-based:

127. Number of orientations per year.. ☐☐

128. Number of inservice and continuing education courses per year .... ☐☐

If academic setting:

129. Number of critical care nursing undergraduate courses per year .... ☐☐

130. Number of critical care nursing graduate courses per year .... ☐☐

131. Number of critical care nursing continuing education courses per year .... ☐☐

If private providers:

132. Number of critical care nursing inservice courses per year.................. ☐☐

133. Number of critical care nursing continuing education courses per year .... ☐☐

Program Formats

134. Rank order the following formats in terms of participant preference (1=most preferred):

Self-instruction . . . . □

Lecture . . . . □

Workshop . . . . □

Group discussion . . . . □

Other (please indicate):_____ . . . . □

Program Evaluation

Frequency
0 does not apply
1 never
2 seldom
3 sometimes
4 frequently
5 always

Usefulness
0 does not apply
1 not useful
2 moderately useful
3 quite useful
4 extremely useful

	Freq.	Use.
135. Institutional providers evaluate critical care education programs they sponsor	□	□
136. Critical care instructors participate in program evaluation	□	□
137. Critical care nurses who are directly involved with patient care participate in the evaluation of critical-care education programs	□	□
138. Critical care nurse managers participate in evaluation of critical care education programs for their staff and other learners	□	□
139. Providers evaluate program effectiveness in meeting learning needs of the critical care nurse	□	□
140. Providers evaluate programs relative to the health needs of the patient populations in critical care areas	□	□
141. Providers evaluate programs relative to the realities of the critical care practice setting	□	□
142. Providers evaluate critical care nursing education programs relative to their administrative framework	□	□
143. Providers evaluate programs relative to the standards of applicable professional accrediting bodies and/or regulatory agencies	□	□

Indicate the frequency with which each of the following features is evaluated in your setting by providers and learners of critical care eduction. Use the following rating scale for frequency:

Frequency
0 not applicable
1 never
2 seldom
3 sometimes
4 frequently
5 always

Feature	A Education Providers	B Learners
144. Relevance and priority of instructional objectives (IO)	☐	☐
145. Behavioral and measurable attributes of IO	☐	☐
146. Consistency and correlation between IO and instructional content	☐	☐
147. Consistency, validity and correlation between IO and evaluation tools used to validate learning acquisition	☐	☐
148. Effectiveness of instructors	☐	☐
149. Quality of instruction	☐	☐
150. Impact of learning environment in facilitating learning	☐	☐

For each of the following statements, indicate both the frequency with which each statement occurs and its usefulness to critical care nursing education activities:

Frequency
0 does not apply
1 never
2 seldom
3 sometimes
4 frequently
5 always

Usefulness
0 does not apply
1 not useful
2 moderately useful
3 quite useful
4 extremely useful

	Freq.	Use.
151. Providers evaluate the program relative to learners' ability to apply learning in critical care nursing practice	☐	☐
152. Providers evaluate the program relative to learners' attainment of instructional objectives	☐	☐
153. Providers evaluate the program relative to the adequacy of resources needed to support the program	☐	☐
154. Providers incorporate both formative and summative evaluations of the program	☐	☐
155. Providers periodically revise programs based on the data contained in the evaluative records	☐	☐

Thank you for your participation in this study. We appreciate your time and efforts in completing this form. Please return the form in the enclosed envelope by the date specified in the cover letter.

___ Appendix C

A NATIONAL SURVEY OF CRITICAL CARE NURSING EDUCATION: FINAL REPORT*

___ Introduction

In 1981 the American Association of Critical-Care Nurses' (AACN) Education Standards Task Force was created and charged with the responsibility for developing the *Educational Standards for Critical Care Nursing.* The Education Standards Task Force completed a literature search in critical care nursing education, designed a conceptual framework and model for the project and refined preliminary drafts of the standards statements. The literature search revealed a virtual void of information characterizing critical care nursing education as it exists in academic, service (health care agency) and private sector settings.

PURPOSE

This investigation was undertaken to gather baseline descriptive information about educational programs offered to critical care nurses. The purpose of the study was to develop a profile or characterization of critical care nursing education in the United States. It was hoped that results would provide a basis upon which to judge the impact of the standards and evaluate the changes in critical care nursing education that will occur over time.

A contract was developed with Assessment Systems, Inc. (ASI) of Philadelphia to conduct the study.

The intent of the Task Force's efforts was to perform a survey to gather data to address the following questions:

1. What is the rationale for providing critical care nursing education in each of its three settings (academic, service, private)?
2. Who are the providers (institutional and individual) of critical care nursing education in each setting? What are their credentials and demographic characteristics? What is their profile?

---

*The survey was conducted, and this report prepared, by Assessment Systems, Inc. (ASI).

3. How is critical care nursing education provided in each setting? What means, methods, techniques and practices are employed in the provision of critical care nursing education? How are programs coordinated and administered?
4. How is critical care nursing education evaluated in each setting?
5. What institutional and professional factors influence critical care nursing education in each setting?
6. Who are the recipients of critical care nursing education in each setting? What are their demographic characteristics? What is their profile?
7. What are the expected outcomes of critical care nursing in each setting?

SURVEY INSTRUMENT DESIGN

Prior to the initiation of this study, the Task Force specified a number of statements grouped around thirteen headings that characterize critical care nursing education programs. The thirteen headings were intended to serve only as a means for logically organizing descriptive statements, not to be viewed as formal standards. The areas for which specific statements were written are:

1. Program Elements
2. Human Resources
3. Financial Resources
4. Material Resources
5. Environmental Resources
6. Assessment of Learning Needs
7. Data Gathering Techniques
8. Resources to Achieve Program Goals
9. Program Goals and Objectives
10. Program Formats
11. Evaluation Strategies
12. Program Implementation
13. Program Evaluation

It was decided by the research team to begin with the Task Force's descriptive statements and to add further statements and questions to cover comprehensively the program dimensions listed above. The wording of each statement was carefully edited to assure that it related to an aspect of an educational program and could be understood as a characteristic of such a program.

Since these statements are characteristics of educational programs, it was considered important to know the frequency with which each element of a program occurs and its perceived usefulness to critical care nursing education activities. The two rating scales specified to assess frequency with which elements occurred and their perceived usefulness are:

Frequency	Usefulness
0 = Does not apply	0 = Does not apply
1 = Never	1 = Not useful
2 = Seldom	2 = Moderately useful
3 = Sometimes	3 = Quite useful
4 = Frequently	4 = Extremely useful
5 = Always	

The actual survey instrument consisted of one hundred fifty-four statements.* Ninety-eight of the statements required respondents to indicate the relative frequency of occurrence of the stated program element within their critical care nursing education program. In addition those same statements were rated as to the respondents' degree of perceived usefulness to critical care nursing education activities. The remaining fifty-six statements required responses to other rating scales or a number or percentage response. Several statements were worded as questions and were structured in such a manner as to require multiple responses by respondents. The presentation of survey findings is ordered in the same sequence as the survey instrument and provides a brief description of the response format. A copy of the survey instrument can be found in Appendix B.

In order to describe respondents who participated in this study, it was necessary to gather data that would outline demographic characteristics. Twelve questions were specified that were considered to be important in describing the group of respondents. These questions were also considered with regard to their possible relationship to respondents' judgments concerning the frequency and usefulness of program characteristics. The twelve demographic variables are:

1. Sex
2. Age
3. Nursing Education
4. Primary Area of Practice
5. Full/Part-time Employment
6. Nonprofit/For-profit Setting
7. Primary Practice Setting
8. Geographic Region
9. Rural/Suburban/Urban Location
10. Years in Critical Care Education
11. Years in Critical Care Nursing
12. Professional Nursing Certifications

PILOT TEST OF SURVEY INSTRUMENT

In order to determine the appropriateness of the survey structure and wording, a small group of critical care nurse educators was identified by the Task Force, and their cooperation in a pilot test was solicited by the chairperson. Ten draft survey forms and instructions were mailed along with the cover letter to be used in the actual study. Each educator was asked to read and react to all aspects of the survey. Of the ten forms mailed, five (50%) were returned. Those survey forms that contained responses to rating scales and questions were reviewed to determine possible problems in the instrument's clarity and intent. In addition comments made by pilot test participants were studied to ascertain the need for additional statements, instructions and clarification. These comments were used by ASI staff in cooperation with the Task Force chairperson to restructure questions and edit statements for greater clarity.

---

*Due to a typographical error (the omission of the number 63), the last item number is 155. However, there are 154 items.

_____ Methodology

The intent of this study was to obtain the judgments of critical care nurse educators with regard to the frequency of occurrence of selected characteristics of educational programs and the usefulness of each to critical care nurse education programs. The overall plan for this investigation was to identify groups of critical care nurse educators and solicit their responses to the survey instrument designed to capture program-related information. The purpose was to provide a description of critical care nurse educators and programs.

RESPONDENTS

To gather data about critical care nurse educators from the educators themselves, it was first necessary to define where such education occurs and who is responsible for these activities. The Task Force initially identified three sources of educational providers of critical care nurse education services:

1. Academic institutions
2. Private providers
3. Service providers

The identification of the population of critical care nurse education programs at academic institutions (group #1 above) was based on a listing of such programs in the National League for Nursing's publication entitled _Master's Education In Nursing: Route to Opportunities in Contemporary Nursing 1985-86_ (NLN, Pub. No. 15-1312; 1985). The private provider category (group #2 above) was defined as those individuals and organizations who have been granted continuing education units (CEU) approval by the American Association of Critical-Care Nurses (AACN). This list, maintained and supplied by the AACN, contains the names of private consultants and a variety of companies.

As defined above, the population of academic institutions and private providers were mailed survey forms addressed to the company or institution in care of the director of critical care nurse education. Where names were available, survey forms were addressed directly to the names provided.

Information about the population of hospitals that provide critical care nurse education services (group #3 above) was not available. It was assumed that hospitals with critical care units (CCU) and/or intensive care units (ICU) would most likely be the institutions that provide for the education of critical care nurses. However, it was not assumed that every hospital with such units would provide critical care nurse education. Based on these assumptions and the objective of gathering information from those individuals responsible for critical care nurse education, a mailing list of hospitals that have either CCUs and/or ICUs was secured (Business Mailers, Inc.; Ridgefield, New Jersey). Letters were addressed and mailed to directors of nursing education requesting the individual responsible for critical care nurse education to agree to participate in the study. This letter came jointly from the president of AACN and the chairperson of the Education Standards Task Force and solicited a professional commitment to respond by a specified date. This mailing to service providers occurred on July 5, 1985 requesting a response within ten days. This response was in the form of a business reply postcard. Of the 4280 hospitals on the purchased mailing list, 1280 responded with a name and address of an individual responsible for critical care education activities.

On August 13th and 14th the actual survey forms were mailed to those individuals who responded to the participation request and to all academic institutions and private providers. The letter covering the survey form requested a response within seventeen days from the mailing date. In order to obtain the research team's anticipated number of respondents to the survey instrument (N = 600), a reminder postcard was sent on September 1, 1985, to all those mailed an original survey form. This card requested those who had not yet responded to do so and thanked those who already had responded. In addition a telephone number was provided for anyone who may have lost the original survey form. The final date for including data in the final statistical analysis was September 18, 1985.

In order to determine whether the respondents who returned their completed survey forms prior to the reminder (N = 512) did not differ demographically from those who returned their forms following the reminder (N = 125), a set of comparisons was undertaken. The frequency distribution of all demographic variables for both sets of respondents was examined. The percentages by category and rank orderings showed no apparent differences.

The results of statistical tests based on the original respondents were compared to the same statistical test results from the second set of respondents. The results of an analysis of variance comparing a sample of seven program elements across classifications of five demographic variables for the original respondents resulted in thirteen significant F-tests. These same comparisons on the second set of respondents resulted in eleven of the original groups' thirteen tests also demonstrating significance. Out of a total of thirty-five comparisons between respondent groups, only two differed in their results. While significant for the original respondent group, the two comparisons missed a significance level for the second group by .0093 and .0043 respectively.

The results of these two efforts demonstrate that the early and later respondents do not differ in their demographic characteristics or their judgments regarding program elements. Each set of respondents can be considered as part of the same group.

The following table is a summary of the responses by provider categories:

	Number mailed	Returned surveys	Percent returned
Academic institution	20	7	35%
Private provider	89	10	11%
Service provider	1,280	616	48%
(setting unknown)		(4)	
TOTALS	1,389	637	46%

Of the hospitals sent participation request forms, 29.9% (N = 1280) had personnel associated in some way with critical care nurse education and had indicated the name of a person who should receive the survey form. The total percent returned (46%) is based on the number mailed to academic institutions, private providers and those service providers who agreed to participate.

DATA ANALYSIS

The data analysis plan for survey results was divided into two parts: (1) respondent characteristics and (2) program characteristics. The first part involved the summarization of the demographic information provided by respondents (see survey instrument design above). Frequency distributions and cross-tabulations with chi-square tests for the twelve demographic variables were planned to describe the respondent group. In addition this analysis would provide information necessary for a determination of whether any regrouping of demographic characteristics prior to performing any group comparisons of program elements would be necessary.

The second effort to summarize survey results focused on comparing respondent judgments of the frequency of occurrence and perceived usefulness of program characteristics. Statistical comparisons were made between categories of respondents on their responses or ratings to program characteristics presented in the survey instrument. A one-way analysis of variance was computed for each of the appropriate items across each classification of respondent. Since no research hypotheses were specified for this investigation, a higher statistical significance level ($p < .01$) was used to identify comparisons to report. Post-hoc analyses (Scheffe) were performed on all statistically significant F-tests with degrees of freedom of two or more.

Where appropriate, means, standard deviations, medians and other statistics are presented to describe respondent assessments of the stated program elements.

——— Results
PART I. RESPONDENT CHARACTERISTICS

The data summarized in this section includes a presentation of the frequencies (F) and percentages (%) of respondents by each of the demographic variables included in the background information section of the survey instrument. In addition cross-tabulations were performed on these variables to better describe respondent characteristics.

Table 1 summarizes the frequencies and percentages for each of the twelve demographic variables.

Simple frequencies and percentages were calculated, contingency tables were constructed and the relationships among demographic variables were tested. Chi-square tests were run on all variables to determine the degree to which observed frequencies differed from what would have been expected based on chance. The following presentation describes the results of those tests with significance levels equal to or greater than .01.

As shown in Table 1, there were more females (N = 593) who responded to this survey than males (N = 43). Table 2 presents the distribution of males and females by age categories. The chi square comparing age with sex indicates that the observed frequences in cells are significantly greater than what would be expected on the basis of chance. An examination of Table 2 shows a large number of females across all age categories while the largest number of males is in the age category of 30-39. There are no males in the 40-49 age category and only one is in the 50+ category.

Table 1 —— A summary of frequencies and related percentages on twelve demographic variables*

	F	%
1. Sex:		
Male	43	6.8
Female	593	93.2
2. Age:		
20-29	100	15.8
30-39	398	62.8
40-49	110	17.4
50+	26	4.1
3. Nursing education (highest level completed):		
(A) AD	69	9.8
Diploma	153	21.7
Bachelor's	236	33.5
Master's	165	23.4
Doctorate	1	.1
(B) Non-nursing		
Bachelor's	49	6.9
Master's	30	4.3
Doctorate	2	.3
4. Primary area of practice:		
Administration		
Director of critical care nursing	91	14.4
Head nurse	120	19.0
Supervisor	75	11.9
Educational		
Director of critical care education	108	17.1
Critical care instructor	154	24.4
Clinical		
Staff nurse	16	2.5
Clinical nurse specialist	59	9.3
Private practice		
Business	4	.6
Continuing nursing education provider	5	.8
Professional nursing association	0	0
5. Employment:		
Part-time	42	6.6
Full-time	592	93.4
6. Primary employment setting:		
Nonprofit	550	87.9
For-profit	76	12.1
7. Primary practice setting:		
Community hospital	517	81.9
University teaching hospital	68	10.8
Military or federal hospital	29	4.6
Number of beds in work setting:		
Fewer than 50	16	4.0
50-99	66	16.5
100-199	82	20.6
200-299	89	22.3
300-399	59	14.8
400+	87	21.8

*Note: The sum of frequencies reported may not total 637 due to information omitted by respondents. Percentages are based on number of valid responses.

Continued.

Table 1 —— A summary of frequencies and related percentages on twelve demographic variables — cont'd

	F	%
7. Primary practice setting — cont'd		
Academic institution	7	1.1
Number of students:		
Fewer than 5,000	5	83.3
5,000-7,999	0	0.0
8,000-10,999	0	0.0
11,000-13,999	0	0.0
14,000-16,999	1	16.7
17,000-19,999	0	0.0
20,000+	0	0.0
	(missing 1 case)	
Business	9	1.4
Number of employees:		
Self employed/solo practice	0	0.0
2-9	4	44.5
10-20	3	33.3
21+	2	22.2
Association	1	.2
Number of employees:		
Fewer than 3	0	0.0
3-29	0	0.0
30-49	0	0.0
50-99	0	0.0
100+	1	100.0
8. In which geographic region do you practice?		
Region 1 (CT, MA, ME, NH, RI, VT)	33	5.2
Region 2 (PA, NJ, NY)	95	15.0
Region 3 (DE, DC, FL, GA, MD, NC, SC, VA, WV)	98	15.5
Region 4 (IL, IN, MI, OH, WI)	123	19.4
Region 5 (AL, KY, MS, TN)	34	5.4
Region 6 (IA, KS, MN, MO, NE, ND, SD)	66	10.4
Region 7 (AR, LA, OK, TX)	52	8.2
Region 8 (AZ, CO, ID, MT, NM, NV, UT, WY)	37	5.8
Region 9 (AK, CA, HI, OR, WA)	95	15.0
9. Which of the following locations best describes your practice area?		
Rural	189	29.5
Suburban	197	31.6
Urban	243	38.9
10. Number of years of experience in critical care education:		
Fewer than 2	134	21.6
2-3	101	16.3
4-5	153	24.7
6-10	149	24.1
11-15	57	9.2
16-20	19	3.1
20+	6	1.0

Table 1 — A summary of frequencies and related percentages on twelve demographic variables — cont'd

	F	%
11. Number of years of experience in critical care nursing:		
Fewer than 2	13	2.1
2-3	24	3.8
4-5	87	13.8
6-10	241	38.2
11-15	191	30.3
16-20	58	9.2
20+	17	2.7
12. Professional nursing certifications held:		
CRNA	3	.9
CCRN	322	92.3
CEN	10	2.9
CNRN	1	.3
CVNS	6	1.7
CNOR	0	0.0
RNC	7	2.0
RNCS	0	0.0

Table 2 — Summary of the relationship between respondents' sex and age

COUNT ROW PCT COL PCT TOT PCT	Sex Male	Sex Female	Row total
20-29	5 5.0 11.6 .8	95 95.0 16.1 15.0	100 15.8
30-39	37 9.3 86.0 5.8	361 90.7 61.1 56.9	398 62.8
40-49		110 100.0 18.6 17.4	110 17.4
50+	1 3.8 2.3 .2	25 96.2 4.2 3.9	26 4.1
Column total	43 6.8	591 93.2	634 100.0

Age

Chi-square	D.F.	Significance
12.83950	3	0.0050

Number of missing observations = 3

The relationship between types of certifications and sex is presented in Table 3. The chi square computed for this comparison is significant beyond $p < .01$. A large proportion (92.2%) of respondents hold the CCRN designation. The variation between the sexes with regard to types of certifications is not a chance occurrence.

Chi-square comparisons for all other demographic variables with sex were not significant.

Table 3 ___ Summary of the relationship between respondents' sex and certifications held

COUNT ROW PCT COL PCT TOT PCT		Sex		Row total
		Male	Female	
CRNA		1 33.3 5.3 .3	2 66.7 .6 .6	3 .9
CCRN		14 4.4 73.7 4.0	307 95.6 93.3 88.2	321 92.2
CEN		1 10.0 5.3 .3	9 90.0 2.7 2.6	10 2.9
CNRN			1 100.0 .3 .3	1 .3
CVNS		2 33.3 10.5 .6	4 66.7 1.2 1.1	6 1.7
RNC		1 14.3 5.3 .3	6 85.7 1.8 1.7	7 2.0
Column total		19 5.5	329 94.5	348 100.0

(Row label: Nursing certifications)

Chi-square	*D.F.*	*Significance*
15.81060	5	0.0074

Number of missing observations = 289

When age of respondent was compared with nursing educational level, a significant relationship was found. The frequencies presented in Table 4 show that the younger respondents have a higher proportion of higher degrees. Approximately forty-three percent (42.8%) of the respondents who hold bachelor's or master's degrees are in the ages 30-39 category.

Only one respondent out of the 391 respondents in the ages 30-39 category holds a doctorate degree. Approximately sixty-three percent (62.9%) of all respondents were in this age category.

Table 4 —— Summary of the relationship between respondents' age and level of education

COUNT ROW PCT COL PCT TOT PCT	20-29	Age 30-39	40-49	50+	Row total
Associate degree	11 15.9 11.0 1.8	46 66.7 11.8 7.4	12 17.4 11.3 1.9		69 11.1
Diploma	14 9.2 14.0 2.3	78 51.0 19.9 12.5	45 29.4 42.5 7.2	16 10.5 64.0 2.6	153 24.6
Bachelor's	55 23.4 55.0 8.8	146 62.1 37.3 23.5	26 11.1 24.5 4.2	8 3.4 32.0 1.3	235 37.8
Master's	20 12.2 20.0 3.2	120 73.2 30.7 19.3	23 14.0 21.7 3.7	1 .6 4.0 .2	164 26.4
Doctorate		1 100.0 .3 .2			1 .2
Column total	100 16.1	391 62.9	106 17.0	25 4.0	622 100.0

Nursing education

Chi-square	D.F.	Significance
63.99320	12	0.0000

Number of missing observations = 15

An examination of area of practice against age is shown in Table 5. Each of the major areas of practice is subdivided into appropriate categories. For purposes of discussion, these four categories are referred to as administrators, educators, clinicians and private providers (see further breakdowns in table headings).

Table 5 shows that approximately forty-six percent (45.7%) of the respondents are in the categories of administration and forty-two percent (41.5%) are classified as educators. There is a large number of young respondents in the administration and educator categories (68.6%).

Table 6 presents the cross-tabulation of age by years of experience in critical care education. The observed differences in the proportion of each group belonging to a particular category did not occur solely by chance.

The 30-39 age group category is disproportionately represented in all categories of critical care education experience. The younger respondents have less experience while the older respondents have more experience.

Table 7 presents age of respondents crossed with years of critical care nursing experience. The significant chi square indicates that the relationship between these two variables is not a chance occurrence. Younger respondents have less experience than do older respondents.

No other variables were shown to have a significant relationship with categories of respondent age.

The comparison of the demographic variable of highest nursing degree of the respondent to other demographic variables resulted in five significant chi-square values at $p < .01$. Table 8 presents the cross-tabulation of highest degree of respondent to indicated area of practice.

An examination of the table indicates that educators report having higher degree levels than do administrators. Forty-nine percent (48.7%) of the administrators have bachelor's and master's degrees compared to seventy-five percent (75.0%) of the educators. The largest percent of associate degree and diploma respondents are in the three categories of administration (65%) followed by educators with ten percent (28.8%). Within the clinical categories the staff nurse responses are more like those of the administrators in that approximately fifty-six percent (56.3%) have associate degrees or diplomas while forty-three percent (43.8%) have bachelor's or master's degrees. Overall the clinical nurse specialist has the largest percentage of higher degree levels with ninety-six percent (96.5%) holding bachelor's or master's degrees. Nearly eighty percent of the clinical nurse specialists (79.3%) hold master's degrees.

The comparison of degree level of respondents to their primary practice setting is presented in Table 9. The community hospital respondents show a larger percentage of associate degrees and diplomas (38.8%) than do any of the other categories of practice setting. The association respondent holds a diploma. In contrast there is a large percentage of respondents who hold master's degrees within the categories of university teaching hospital (40.9%), military hospital (55.2%), academic institution (42.9%) and business (71.4%).

Table 5 ___ Summary of the relationship between respondents' age and area of practice

COUNT ROW PCT COL PCT TOT PCT		Age				Row total
		20-29	30-39	40-49	50+	
Administration	Director of critical care nursing	13 14.3 13.0 2.1	49 53.8 12.4 7.8	24 26.4 22.4 3.8	5 5.5 20.0 .8	91 14.5
	Head nurse	16 13.3 16.0 2.6	81 67.5 20.6 12.9	16 13.3 15.0 2.6	7 5.8 28.0 1.1	120 19.2
	Supervisor	12 16.0 12.0 1.9	36 48.0 9.1 5.8	22 29.3 20.6 3.5	5 6.7 20.0 .8	75 12.0
Education	Director of critical care education	20 18.9 20.0 3.2	69 65.1 17.5 11.0	14 13.2 13.1 2.2	3 2.8 12.0 .5	106 16.9
	Critical care instructor	28 18.2 28.0 4.5	105 68.2 26.6 16.8	18 11.7 16.8 2.9	3 1.9 12.0 .5	154 24.6
Clinical	Staff nurse	6 37.5 6.0 1.0	7 43.8 1.8 1.1	2 12.5 1.9 .3	1 6.3 4.0 .2	16 2.6
	Clinical nurse specialist	5 8.5 5.0 .8	44 74.6 11.2 7.0	9 15.3 8.4 1.4	1 1.7 4.0 .2	59 9.4
Private practice	Continuing nursing education provider		3 60.0 .8 .5	2 40.0 1.9 .3		5 .8
	Column total	100 16.0	394 62.9	107 17.1	25 4.0	626 100.0

Chi-square	D.F.	Significance
40.04191	21	0.0073

Number of missing observations = 11

Table 6 — Summary of the relationship between respondents' age and years of critical care education experience

| | | Age | | | Row |
COUNT ROW PCT COL PCT TOT PCT	20-29	30-39	40-49	50+	total
<2	49 36.6 50.5 8.0	72 53.7 18.5 11.7	12 9.0 11.3 1.9	1 .7 4.2 .2	134 21.8
2-3	20 20.2 20.6 3.2	71 71.7 18.3 11.5	7 7.1 6.6 1.1	1 1.0 4.2 .2	99 16.1
4-5	18 11.8 18.6 2.9	115 75.2 29.6 18.7	18 11.8 17.0 2.9	2 1.3 8.3 .3	153 24.8
6-10	10 6.7 10.3 1.6	102 68.5 26.2 16.6	29 19.5 27.4 4.7	8 5.4 33.3 1.3	149 24.2
11-15		27 48.2 6.9 4.4	22 39.3 20.8 3.6	7 12.5 29.2 1.1	56 9.1
16-20		2 10.5 .5 .3	13 68.4 12.3 2.1	4 21.1 16.7 .6	19 3.1
20+			5 83.3 4.7 .8	1 16.7 4.2 .2	6 1.0
Column total	97 15.7	389 63.1	106 17.2	24 3.9	616 100.0

Years of experience in critical care education

Chi-square	D.F.	Significance
192.30558	18	0.0

Number of missing observations = 21

Table 7 —— Summary of the relationship between respondents' age and years of critical care nursing experience

COUNT ROW PCT COL PCT TOT PCT	Age				Row total
	20-29	30-39	40-49	50+	
<2	2 15.4 2.0 .3	9 69.2 2.3 1.4	2 15.4 1.8 .3		13 2.1
2-3	8 33.3 8.1 1.3	14 58.3 3.6 2.2	2 8.3 1.8 .3		24 3.8
4-5	34 39.5 34.3 5.4	45 52.3 11.5 7.2	6 7.0 5.5 1.0	1 1.2 3.8 .2	86 13.7
6-10	55 22.8 55.6 8.8	160 66.4 40.7 25.5	24 10.0 21.8 3.8	2 .8 7.7 .3	241 38.4
11-15		142 74.7 36.1 22.6	35 18.4 31.8 5.6	13 6.8 50.0 2.1	190 30.3
16-20		23. 39.7 5.9 3.7	29 50.0 26.4 4.6	6 10.3 23.1 1.0	58 9.2
20+			12 75.0 10.9 1.9	4 25.0 15.4 .6	16 2.5
Column total	99 15.8	393 62.6	110 17.5	26 4.1	628 100.0

Years of experience in critical care nursing

Chi-square	*D.F*	*Significance*
221.32009	18	0.0

Number of missing observations = 9

Table 8 — Summary of the relationship between respondents' level of education and area of practice

COUNT ROW PCT COL PCT TOT PCT	Nursing education					Row total
	Associate degree	Diploma	Bachelor's	Master's	Doctorate	
Administration — Director of critical care nursing	17 19.1 24.6 2.8	21 23.6 14.2 3.4	30 33.7 12.7 4.9	21 23.6 12.9 3.4		89 14.4
Head nurse	27 22.7 39.1 4.4	44 37.0 29.7 7.1	40 33.6 16.9 6.5	8 6.7 4.9 1.3		119 19.3
Supervisor	6 8.2 8.7 1.0	27 37.0 18.2 4.4	31 42.5 13.1 5.0	8 11.0 4.9 1.3	1 1.4 100.0 .2	73 11.8
Education — Director of critical care education	7 6.7 10.1 1.1	17 16.2 11.5 2.8	43 41.0 18.2 7.0	38 36.2 23.3 6.2		105 17.0
Critical care instructor	6 3.9 8.7 1.0	34 22.2 23.0 5.5	76 49.7 32.2 12.3	37 24.2 22.7 6.0		153 24.8
Clinical — Staff nurse	5 31.3 7.2 .8	4 25.0 2.7 .6	6 37.5 2.5 1.0	1 6.3 .6 .2		16 2.6
Clinical nurse specialist	1 1.7 1.4 .2	1 1.7 .7 .2	10 17.2 4.2 1.6	46 79.3 28.2 7.5		58 9.4
Private practice — Continuing nursing education provider				4 100.0 2.5 .6		4 .6
Column total	69 11.2	148 24.0	236 38.2	163 26.4	1 .2	617 100.0

Chi-square	*D.F.*	*Significance*
192.05231	28	0.0

Number of missing observations = 20

Table 9 —— Summary of the relationship between respondents' level of education and practice setting

COUNT ROW PCT COL PCT TOT PCT	Nursing education					Row total
	Associate degree	Diploma	Bachelor's	Master's	Doctorate	
Community hospital	63 12.4 92.6 10.2	134 26.4 89.3 21.7	196 38.6 83.8 31.7	114 22.4 69.1 18.4	1 .2 100.0 .2	508 82.2
University teaching hospital	5 7.6 7.4 .8	6 9.1 4.0 1.0	28 42.4 12.0 4.5	27 40.9 16.4 4.4		66 10.7
Military hospital		5 17.2 3.3 .8	8 27.6 3.4 1.3	16 55.2 9.7 2.6		29 4.7
Academic institution		2 28.6 1.3 .3	2 28.6 .9 .3	3 42.9 1.8 .5		7 1.1
Business		2 28.6 1.3 .3		5 71.4 3.0 .8		7 1.1
Association		1 100.0 .7 .2				1 .2
Column total	68 11.0	150 24.3	234 37.9	165 26.7	1 .2	618 100.0

Practice setting

Chi-square	D.F.	Significance
44.79444	20	0.0012

Number of missing observations = 19

Table 10 —— Summary of the relationship between respondents' level of education and location of practice

COUNT ROW PCT COL PCT TOT PCT	Associate degree	Diploma	Bachelor's	Master's	Doctorate	Row total
			Nursing education			
Rural	35	64	66	17	1	183
	19.1	35.0	36.1	9.3	.5	29.9
	52.2	44.1	28.0	10.4	100.0	
	5.7	10.5	10.8	2.8	.2	
Suburban	16	47	73	57		193
	8.3	24.4	37.8	29.5		31.5
	23.9	32.4	30.9	35.0		
	2.6	7.7	11.9	9.3		
Urban	16	34	97	89		236
	6.8	14.4	41.1	37.7		38.6
	23.9	23.4	41.1	54.6		
	2.6	5.6	15.8	14.5		
Column total	67	145	236	163	1	612
	10.9	23.7	38.6	26.6	.2	100.0

(Practice location — left axis label spanning Rural, Suburban, Urban)

Chi-square	D.F.	Significance
69.83659	8	0.0000

Number of missing observations = 25

An examination of the distribution of respondent degree level by location (rural, suburban, urban) is presented in Table 10. Within the rural location category, approximately forty-five percent (45.4%) of the respondents have bachelor's and master's degrees. Sixty-seven percent (67.3%) of the respondents from suburban locations and seventy-nine percent (78.8%) of the respondents from urban locations have bachelor's and master's degrees. The urban areas have the highest concentration of bachelor's and master's degree respondents followed by the suburban location: rural locations have almost fifty percent fewer respondents with these degrees.

A comparison of respondents' highest degree level with critical care nursing education experience shows that the greatest experience levels are held by those respondents with diplomas. Table 11 presents this data and shows that respondents with bachelor's and master's degrees tend to have more experience than do associate degrees or diploma respondents. At the lower experience levels there tends to be nearly twice the number of bachelor's and master's degrees than associate degrees and diplomas.

Thirty-nine percent (38.6%) of the respondents have fewer than four years of experience in critical care nursing education, while almost half (48.4%) of the respondents have between four and ten years of experience.

Table 11 —— Summary of the relationship between respondents' level of education and years of critical care education experience

COUNT ROW PCT COL PCT TOT PCT	Nursing education					Row total
	Associate degree	Diploma	Bachelor's	Master's	Doctorate	
<2	22 16.4 32.8 3.6	25 18.7 17.2 4.1	61 45.5 26.4 10.1	26 19.4 16.0 4.3		134 22.1
2-3	8 8.0 11.9 1.3	20 20.0 13.8 3.3	47 47.0 20.3 7.8	25 25.0 15.4 4.1		100 16.5
4-5	20 13.3 29.9 3.3	23 15.3 15.9 3.8	59 39.3 25.5 9.7	48 32.0 29.6 7.9		150 24.8
6-10	12 8.4 17.9 2.0	42 29.4 29.0 6.9	44 30.8 19.0 7.3	45 31.5 27.8 7.4		143 23.6
11-15	4 7.3 6.0 .7	23 41.8 15.9 3.8	15 27.3 6.5 2.5	12 21.8 7.4 2.0	1 1.8 100.0 .2	55 9.1
16-20	1 5.6 1.5 .2	7 38.9 4.8 1.2	4 22.2 1.7 .7	6 33.3 3.7 1.0		18 3.0
20+		5 83.3 3.4 .8	1 16.7 .4 .2			6 1.0
Column total	67 11.1	145 23.9	231 38.1	162 26.7	1 .2	606 100.0

Chi-square   *D.F.*   *Significance*

61.98073   24   0.0000

Number of missing observations = 31

Table 12 presents respondent degree level broken down by years of critical care nursing experience. In contrast to Table 11, only six percent (6%) of the respondents have fewer than three years of experience in critical care nursing. Fifty-two percent (52.4%) have between four and ten years of experience in critical care nursing.

The largest percentage of respondents in the six to fifteen years of experience categories (67.1%) have bachelor's and master's degrees while only thirty-three percent (32.9%) within the same experience categories hold associate degrees and diplomas. At the higher levels of experience (16-20+ years), there are no differences in percent of degrees by bachelor's and master's degree and associate degree and diploma.

The following information shows the results of comparisons for categories of area of practice and six demographic variables. The first cross-tabulation compared the categories of areas of practice with employment status (part-time/full time). Ninety-three percent of the respondents were full-time employees with the largest number (22.8%) employed as critical care instructors. The second largest percentage of full-time employee respondents (19.7%) are in the head nurse category under administration. Forty percent (40.1%) and forty-seven percent (47.5%) of the respondents who work full time are instructors and administrators respectively. Forty-seven percent (47.6%) of the respondents who are part-time employees are classified as instructors.

When area of practice is cross-tabulated with whether the respondent's primary employment setting is nonprofit or for-profit, a significant chi square is obtained. Forty-three percent (43.9%) of the respondents from nonprofit settings are in the administration category and the same percentage are classified as educators. Of the respondents from for-profit settings, fifty-eight percent (58.3%) are in administration and twenty-five (25%) are classified as educators.

Table 13 presents area of practice compared to primary practice setting. Ninety-eight percent (97.9%) of the respondents were from community, university or military hospitals with a small percentage from academic institutions, private businesses and associations (2.1%).

Twenty-three percent (23.6%) of the community hospital respondents indicated that they were instructors. Within the university hospital setting, the title of instructor was most frequently reported (32.4%) followed by director of critical care education (23.5%). The titles of head nurse (17.6%) and clinical nurse specialist (13.2%) were frequently reported by respondents from university hospitals. Similar to the university hospital results, respondents from the military hospitals reported most frequently the classifications of head nurse (37.9%), instructor (27.6%) and clinical nurse specialist (13.8%).

The comparison of area of practice with locations is presented in Table 14. The observed differences in the proportion of each area of practice as compared to location did not occur solely by chance.

There is a larger proportion of administrative respondents (72.5%) from the rural category as compared to suburban (42.4%) or urban (28.1%). The inverse of this relationship is true for educators. Rural educators account for twenty-one percent (20.8%), suburban educators for forty-six percent (45.9%) and urban educators account for fifty-three percent (53.2%). Sixteen percent (16.3%) of the urban respondents reported themselves as clinical nurse specialists.

Table 12 —— Summary of the relationship between respondents' level of education and years of critical care nursing experience

COUNT ROW PCT COL PCT TOT PCT	Nursing education					Row total
	Associate degree	Diploma	Bachelor's	Master's	Doctorate	
<2	4 30.8 5.9 .6	2 15.4 1.3 .3	4 30.8 1.7 .6	3 23.1 1.8 .5		13 2.1
2-3	5 21.7 7.4 .8	4 17.4 2.7 .6	10 43.5 4.3 1.6	4 17.4 2.4 .6		23 3.7
4-5	20 23.3 29.4 3.2	7 8.1 4.7 1.1	43 50.0 18.3 7.0	16 18.6 9.7 2.6		86 13.9
6-10	26 10.9 38.2 4.2	53 22.3 35.6 8.6	93 39.1 39.6 15.0	66 27.7 40.0 10.7		238 38.5
11-15	11 5.9 16.2 1.8	50 26.6 33.6 8.1	67 35.6 28.5 10.8	60 31.9 36.4 9.7		188 30.4
16-20	2 3.6 2.9 .3	25 45.5 16.8 4.0	16 29.1 6.8 2.6	11 20.0 6.7 1.8	1 1.8 100.0 .2	55 8.9
20+		8 53.3 5.4 1.3	2 13.3 .9 .3	5 33.3 3.0 .8		15 2.4
Column total	68 11.0	149 24.1	235 38.0	165 26.7	1 .2	618 100.0

Chi-square   *D.F.*   *Significance*

77.97279   24   0.0000

Number of missing observations = 19

Years of experience in critical care nursing

Table 13 — Summary of the relationship between respondents' area of practice and practice setting

| | Administration | | | Education | | Clinical | | Private practice | |
| | Director of critical care nursing | Head nurse | Supervisor | Director of critical care education | Critical care instructor | Staff nurse | Clinical nurse specialist | Continuing nursing education providers | Row total |
COUNT / ROW PCT / COL PCT / TOT PCT									
Community hospital	86 / 16.8 / 94.5 / 13.8	94 / 18.4 / 79.7 / 15.1	66 / 12.9 / 90.4 / 10.6	86 / 16.8 / 80.4 / 13.8	121 / 23.6 / 79.1 / 19.5	14 / 2.7 / 87.5 / 2.3	45 / 8.8 / 76.3 / 7.2		512 / 82.3
University teaching hospital	4 / 5.9 / 4.4 / .6	12 / 17.6 / 10.2 / 1.9	4 / 5.9 / 5.5 / .6	16 / 23.5 / 15.0 / 2.6	22 / 32.4 / 14.4 / 3.5	1 / 1.5 / 6.3 / .2	9 / 13.2 / 15.3 / 1.4		68 / 10.9
Military hospital	1 / 3.4 / 1.1 / .2	11 / 37.9 / 9.3 / 1.8	3 / 10.3 / 4.1 / .5	1 / 3.4 / .9 / .2	8 / 27.6 / 5.2 / 1.3	1 / 3.4 / 6.3 / .2	4 / 13.8 / 6.8 / .6		29 / 4.7

Practice setting

Practice setting

	91 14.6	118 19.0	73 11.7	107 17.2	153 24.6	16 2.6	59 9.5	5 .8	622 100.0
Academic institution		1 14.3 .8 .2		3 42.9 2.8 .5	2 28.6 1.3 .3		1 14.3 1.7 .2		7 1.1
Business								5 100.0 100.0 .8	5 .8
Association				1 100.0 .9 .2					1 .2
Column total	91 14.6	118 19.0	73 11.7	107 17.2	153 24.6	16 2.6	59 9.5	5 .8	622 100.0

Chi-square	D.F.	Significance
656.79496	35	0.0000

Number of missing observations = 15

Table 14 — Summary of the relationship between respondents' area of practice and location of practice

COUNT / ROW PCT / COL PCT / TOT PCT

Practice location	Administration			Education		Clinical		Private practice	Row total
	Director of critical care nursing	Head nurse	Supervisor	Director of critical care education	Critical care instructor	Staff nurse	Clinical nurse specialist	Continuing nursing education providers	
Rural	41 22.5 45.1 6.6	51 28.0 43.6 8.3	40 22.0 54.1 6.5	19 10.4 18.3 3.1	19 10.4 12.6 3.1	8 4.4 50.0 1.3	4 2.2 6.8 .6		182 29.5
Suburban	30 15.3 33.0 4.9	36 18.4 30.8 5.8	17 8.7 23.0 2.8	32 16.3 30.8 5.2	58 29.6 38.4 9.4	6 3.1 37.5 1.0	16 8.2 27.1 2.6	1 .5 20.0 .2	196 31.8
Urban	20 8.4 22.0 3.2	30 12.6 25.6 4.9	17 7.1 23.0 2.8	53 22.2 51.0 8.6	74 31.0 49.0 12.0	2 .8 12.5 .3	39 16.3 66.1 6.3	4 1.7 80.0 .6	239 38.7
Column total	91 14.7	117 19.0	74 12.0	104 16.9	151 24.5	16 2.6	59 9.6	5 .8	617 100.0

D.F.   Significance

14   0.0000

Number of missing observations = 20

Table 15 presents the cross-tabulation of area of practice with years of critical care education experience. In the categories up to ten years of critical care education experience, there are in general more instructors of critical care than any other category of practice. At the higher levels of experience (11-20+ years), the head nurse and supervisor titles occur more frequently.

In general respondents in the three categories of administration have more critical care nursing education experience than do respondents in any of the other categories of practice.

In comparing area of practice with respondents' years of critical care nursing experience, sixty-nine percent (68.8%) of all respondents have between six and fifteen years of experience. Of this group of respondents, forty-three percent (43.4%) are classified in administration, forty-three percent (43.5%) are in education and twelve percent (12%) are in the clinical categories. Table 16 presents the cross-tabulation of these data.

A review of Table 16 shows that there are few respondents with fewer than three years of critical care nursing experience (6%).

An exploration of the relationship between years of critical care nursing experience and the respondents' primary employment setting is presented in Table 17.

Eighty-eight percent (87.8%) of the respondents are employed by nonprofit organizations. The largest percentage of respondents from nonprofit settings (37.4%) and from for-profit settings (39.5%) have between six and ten years of experience. Those from for-profit settings have more experience (48.6% in the 11-20+ years category) than the nonprofit respondents (41.7%).

Table 18 presents the relationship between primary practice setting and hospital size. The largest number of respondents from community hospitals are from hospitals in the 200-299-bed category (23.9%) followed closely by the 100-199-bed category.

Fifty-five percent (55.8%) of the respondents from university hospitals indicate that the number of beds in their setting is more than four hundred while forty-three percent (42.9%) of those from military hospitals and only sixteen percent (15.6%) of those in community hospitals are of that size. Community hospital respondents are from hospitals ranging from fewer than 50 beds (4.6%) to more than 400 beds (15.6%). Like respondents from community hospitals, those from military hospitals indicate a range of hospital sizes. Seven percent (7.2%) of the military hospitals have fewer than 99 beds.

An examination of the distribution of primary practice setting by location also results in a significant chi-square value. Table 19 presents the results of this comparison. The respondents are almost evenly split across rural (29.6%), suburban (31.4%) and urban (39.1%) locations with the urban location showing a slightly higher percentage of respondents. There were slightly more community hospitals in rural settings (34.1%) as compared to suburban (32.9%) and urban (32.9%). In contrast the university hospitals are predominantly urban (76.5%) as are the military hospitals (46.4%) and businesses (87.5%). The academic setting is evenly split between urban and suburban locations at forty-three percent (42.9%).

Table 15 — Summary of the relationship between respondents' area of practice and years of critical care education experience

COUNT ROW PCT COL PCT TOT PCT	Administration			Education		Clinical		Private practice	Row total
	Director of critical care nursing	Head nurse	Supervisor	Director of critical care education	Critical care instructor	Staff nurse	Clinical nurse specialist	Continuing nursing education providers	
<2	17 12.7 20.0 2.8	31 23.1 27.7 5.1	8 6.0 10.8 1.3	27 20.1 25.2 4.4	36 26.9 23.4 5.9	6 4.5 42.9 1.0	8 6.0 13.6 1.3	1 .7 20.0 .2	134 22.0
2-3	9 9.0 10.8 1.5	10 10.0 8.9 1.6	15 15.0 20.3 2.5	19 19.0 17.8 3.1	34 34.0 22.1 5.6	1 1.0 7.1 .2	12 12.0 20.3 2.0		100 16.4
4-5	27 18.0 31.8 4.4	20 13.3 17.9 3.3	19 12.7 25.7 3.1	22 14.7 20.6 3.6	40 26.7 26.0 6.6	5 3.3 35.7 .8	17 11.3 28.8 2.8		150 24.6
6-10	19 13.1 22.4 3.1	30 20.7 26.8 4.9	12 8.3 16.2 2.0	29 20.0 27.1 4.8	36 24.8 23.4 5.9	1 .7 7.1 .2	17 11.7 28.8 2.8	1 .7 20.0 .2	145 23.8

Years of experience in critical care education

Years of experience in critical care education

									Row total
11-15	8 14.0 9.4 1.3	16 28.1 14.3 2.6	14 24.6 18.9 2.3	6 10.5 5.6 1.0	7 12.3 4.5 1.1	1 1.8 7.1 .2	4 7.0 6.8 .7	1 1.8 20.0 .2	57 9.3
16-20	5 26.3 5.9 .8	3 15.8 2.7 .5	5 26.3 6.8 .8	3 15.8 2.8 .5			1 5.3 1.7 .2	2 10.5 40.0 .3	19 3.1
20+		2 40.0 1.8 .3	1 20.0 1.4 .2	1 20.0 .9 .2	1 20.0 .6 .2				5 .8
Column total	85 13.9	112 18.4	74 12.1	107 17.5	154 25.2	14 2.3	59 9.7	5 .8	610 100.0

Chi-square	*D.F.*	*Significance*	*Min E.F.*	*Cells with E.F. <5*
87.41065	42	0.0000	0.041	26 OF 56 (46.4%)

Number of missing observations = 27

Table 16 — Summary of the relationship between respondents' area of practice and years of critical care nursing experience

Years of experience in critical care nursing	COUNT / ROW PCT / COL PCT / TOT PCT	Administration: Director of critical care nursing	Head nurse	Supervisor	Education: Director of critical care education	Critical care instructor	Clinical: Staff nurse	Clinical nurse specialist	Private practice: Continuing nursing education providers	Row total
<2			4 / 30.8 / 3.4 / .6	3 / 23.1 / 4.1 / .5	2 / 15.4 / 1.9 / .3	1 / 7.7 / .6 / .2	1 / 7.7 / 6.3 / .2	1 / 7.7 / 1.7 / .2	1 / 7.7 / 20.0 / .2	13 / 2.1
2-3		3 / 12.5 / 3.3 / .5	2 / 8.3 / 1.7 / .3	5 / 20.8 / 6.8 / .8	8 / 33.3 / 7.5 / 1.3	5 / 20.8 / 3.2 / .8	1 / 4.2 / 6.3 / .2			24 / 3.9
4-5		12 / 14.1 / 13.2 / 1.9	22 / 25.9 / 18.8 / 3.5	8 / 9.4 / 10.8 / 1.3	15 / 17.6 / 14.2 / 2.4	17 / 20.0 / 11.0 / 2.7	4 / 4.7 / 25.0 / .6	7 / 8.2 / 11.9 / 1.1		85 / 13.7
6-10		39 / 16.4 / 42.9 / 6.3	40 / 16.8 / 34.2 / 6.4	21 / 8.8 / 28.4 / 3.4	42 / 17.6 / 39.6 / 6.8	69 / 29.0 / 44.8 / 11.1	7 / 2.9 / 43.8 / 1.1	19 / 8.0 / 32.2 / 3.1	1 / .4 / 20.0 / .2	238 / 38.3

Years of experience in critical care nursing

									Row total
11-15	25 13.2 27.5 4.0	39 20.5 33.3 6.3	23 12.1 31.1 3.7	24 12.6 22.6 3.9	51 26.8 33.1 8.2	3 1.6 18.8 .5	24 12.6 40.7 3.9	1 .5 20.0 .2	190 30.5
16-20	12 21.8 13.2 1.9	8 14.5 6.8 1.3	8 14.5 10.8 1.3	10 18.2 9.4 1.6	9 16.4 5.8 1.4		7 12.7 11.9 1.1	1 1.8 20.0 .2	55 8.8
20+		2 11.8 1.7 .3	6 35.3 8.1 1.0	5 29.4 4.7 .8	2 11.8 1.3 .3		1 5.9 1.7 .2	1 5.9 20.0 .2	17 2.7
Column total	91 14.6	117 18.8	74 11.9	106 17.0	154 24.8	16 2.6	59 9.5	5 .8	622 100.0

Chi-square	D.F.	Significance	Min E.F.	Cells with E.F. <5
68.85252	42	0.0056	0.105	30 OF 56 (53.6%)

Number of missing observations = 15

Table 17 —— Summary of the relationship between respondents' employment setting and years of critical care nursing experience

COUNT ROW PCT COL PCT TOT PCT	Employment setting		Row total
	Nonprofit	For-profit	
<2	13 100.0 2.4 2.1		13 2.1
2-3	22 91.7 4.0 3.5	2 8.3 2.6 .3	24 3.8
4-5	79 91.9 14.4 12.7	7 8.1 9.2 1.1	86 13.8
6-10	205 87.2 37.4 32.9	30 12.8 39.5 4.8	235 37.7
11-15	170 89.0 31.0 27.2	21 11.0 27.6 3.4	191 30.6
16-20	43 74.1 7.8 6.9	15 25.9 19.7 2.4	58 9.3
20+	16 94.1 2.9 2.6	1 5.9 1.3 .2	17 2.7
Column total	548 87.8	76 12.2	624 100.0

Years of experience in critical care nursing

Chi-square	D.F.	Significance
14.55527	6	0.0240

Number of missing observations = 13

Table 18 —— Summary of the relationship between respondents' practice setting and hospital size

COUNT ROW PCT COL PCT TOT PCT	Practice setting Community hospital	University teaching hosp.	Military hospital	Row total
<50	15 93.8 4.6 3.8		1 6.3 3.6 .3	16 4.0
50-99	62 93.9 19.0 15.6	3 4.5 7.0 .8	1 1.5 3.6 .3	66 16.6
100-199	74 91.4 22.7 18.6	2 2.5 4.7 .5	5 6.2 17.9 1.3	81 20.4
200-299	78 88.6 23.9 19.6	7 8.0 16.3 1.8	3 3.4 10.7 .8	88 22.2
300-399	46 78.0 14.1 11.6	7 11.9 16.3 1.8	6 10.2 21.4 1.5	59 14.9
400+	51 58.6 15.6 12.8	24 27.6 55.8 6.0	12 13.8 42.9 3.0	87 21.9
Column total	326 82.1	43 10.8	28 7.1	397 100.0

Hospital size (beds) (row label on the left margin)

Chi-square	*D.F.*	*Significance*
52.35368	10	0.0000

Number of missing observations = 240

Table 19 —— Summary of the relationship between respondents' practice setting and location of practice

COUNT ROW PCT COL PCT TOT PCT	Practice setting						Row total
	Community hospital	University teaching hospital	Military hospital	Academic institution	Business	Association	
Rural	174 94.6 34.1 28.0	4 2.2 5.9 .6	5 2.7 17.9 .8	1 .5 14.3 .2			184 29.6
Suburban	168 86.2 32.9 27.0	12 6.2 17.6 1.9	10 5.1 35.7 1.6	3 1.5 42.9 .5	1 .5 12.5 .2	1 .5 100.0 .2	195 31.4
Urban	168 69.1 32.9 27.0	52 21.4 76.5 8.4	13 5.3 46.4 2.1	3 1.2 42.9 .5	7 2.9 87.5 1.1		243 39.1
Column total	510 82.0	68 10.9	28 4.5	7 1.1	8 1.3	1 .2	622 100.0

(Practice location — row label)

Chi-square	*D.F.*	*Significance*	*Min E.F.*	*Cells with E.F. <5*
63.19367	10	0.0000	0.296	9 OF 18 (50.0%)

Number of missing observations = 15

The final cross-tabulation of the demographic variables compares respondent experience in critical care education with critical care nursing experience. Table 20 presents the results of this cross-tabulation.

Two percent (2.1%) of the respondents indicated that they have more experience in teaching critical care nursing than experience in critical care nursing. Twenty-four percent (24.0%) of the respondents indicated equal levels of education and nursing experience. Seventy-four percent (73.9%) of the respondents indicated they had more experience in critical care nursing than in critical care education. The largest number of respondents indicated that they had 6-10 years of critical care nursing experience and 4-5 years of critical care education experience.

Table 20 —— Summary of the relationship between respondents' years of critical care education experience and years of critical care nursing experience

COUNT ROW PCT COL PCT TOT PCT	<2	2-3	4-5	6-10	11-15	16-20	20+	Row total
<2	10 76.9 7.5 1.6	2 15.4 2.0 .3		1 7.7 .7 .2				13 2.1
2-3	17 70.8 12.7 2.8	3 12.5 3.0 .5	2 8.3 1.3 .3	2 8.2 1.3 .3				24 3.9
4-5	35 40.7 26.1 5.7	24 27.9 23.8 3.9	23 26.7 15.1 3.7	4 4.7 2.7 .6				86 13.9
6-10	54 22.9 40.3 8.7	47 19.9 46.5 7.6	74 31.4 48.7 12.0	61 25.8 40.9 9.9				236 38.2
11-15	16 8.6 11.9 2.6	19 10.3 18.8 3.1	48 25.9 31.6 7.8	65 35.1 43.6 10.5	36 19.5 63.2 5.8		1 .5 16.7 .2	185 29.9
16-20	2 3.5 1.5 .3	6 10.5 5.9 1.0	5 8.8 3.3 .8	13 22.8 8.7 2.1	17 29.8 29.8 2.8	13 22.8 68.4 2.1	1 1.8 16.7 .2	57 9.2
20+				3 17.6 2.0 .5	4 23.5 7.0 .6	6 35.3 31.6 1.0	4 23.5 66.7 .6	17 2.8
Column total	134 21.7	101 16.3	152 24.6	149 24.1	57 9.2	19 3.1	6 1.0	618 100.0

Years of experience in critical care education (column headings); Years of experience in critical care nursing (row headings)

Chi-square	D.F.	Significance	Min E.F.	Cells with E.F. <5
475.22341	36	0.0000	0.126	24 OF 49 (49.0%)

Number of missing observations = 19

PART II. PROGRAM CHARACTERISTICS

The following presentation shows the results of comparing the mean ratings of respondents to statements of program characteristics. In this section of the survey analysis, the attempt was to determine whether the mean ratings of program elements by classes of respondents differ to a greater degree than would be expected on the basis of chance. There were one hundred fifty-five statements descriptive of educational programs.

Respondents' ratings of program characteristics, grouped by six demographic variables, were compared using analysis of variance techniques. The six key respondent variables and the number of subcategories of each are presented below:

1. Age (3)
2. Years providing critical care education (5)
3. Area of practice (4)
4. Location (3)
5. Years of critical care nursing experience (5)
6. Hospital size (4)

A one-way analysis of variance was performed comparing respondent ratings of frequency of occurrence and usefulness of each program characteristic across subcategories of each variable presented above. A post-hoc analysis was performed on all statistically significant F-tests. Only those overall F-tests with p values less than .01 and significant Scheffe comparisons are summarized and presented in this report. The number presented after each description of a program characteristic is the question number of that characteristic in the original survey form and is used here to facilitate locating the specific variables in tables.

Respondents' age. Comparison of mean ratings of each program characteristic by three categories of age (20-29, 30-39, 40+) resulted in significant differences between only two program characteristics. Table 21 presents the means and standard deviations by age category, the degrees of freedom and the F values for the dependent variable of percentage estimates.

When asked what percent of instructors meet the nursing practice standards of the critical care unit in their area of teaching assignment (36), each age group of respondent differed significantly in their ratings. The older the respondent, the lower the rating of the percent of instructors who meet practice standards. The 20-29 age group indicated that on the average ninety-five percent (94.88%) meet the standard while the 40+ group's average percentage was seventy-six (76.36%).

The judged percentage of instructors demonstrating competence in the application of nursing and scientific concepts and principles to care of the critically ill patient (37) was again higher for the youngest group (94.46%) than the 40+ group (81.81%). There was no difference between the 20-29 group and the 30-39 group of respondents on this program characteristic.

Respondents' years of experience in critical care education. One program characteristic was rated differently by respondents with different years of experience in critical care education relative to its frequency of occurrence. Seven differences were identified relative to respondent ratings of the usefulness of program characteristics.

Table 21 — Summary of significant differences across age categories on percent

Program characteristics	20-29 N = 88		30-39 N = 321		40+ N = 100		DF	F*
	X	SD	X	SD	X	SD		
(36) What percent of instructors meet the nursing practice standards of the critical care unit in their area of teaching assignment?	94.88	16.02	89.23	26.37	76.36	39.14	2	9.10
(37) What percent of instructors demonstrate competence in the application of nursing and scientific concepts and principles to care of the critically ill patient?	94.46	7.88	92.59	21.64	81.81	35.08	2	9.36

*All significant at P ≤.01

Table 22 —— Summary of significant differences across categories of years of experience in critical care education for frequency of occurrence of program characteristics

Program characteristics	<2 N = 134		2-3 N = 101		4-5 N = 155		6-10 N = 149		11+ N = 82		DF	F*
	X	SD	X	SD	X	SD	X	SD	X	SD		
(72) Providers assess the validity and reliability of methods used for collection of assessment data prior to data analysis	2.91	1.14	2.86	1.13	3.16	.96	3.02	1.14	3.44	1.07	4	3.74

*All significant at P ≤ .01
Frequency rating scale:
0 = Does not apply   2 = Seldom   4 = Frequently
1 = Never   3 = Sometimes   5 = Always

Table 23 —— Summary of significant differences across categories of years of experience in critical care education for usefulness of program characteristics

Program characteristics	<2 N = 134		2-3 N = 101		4-5 N = 163		6-10 N = 149		11+ N = 82		DF	F*
	X	SD	X	SD	X	SD	X	SD	X	SD		
(59) Physical facilities are conducive to attainment of program goals and instructional objectives	3.23	.91	2.93	.90	3.27	.75	3.32	.80	3.40	.71	4	4.33
(60) Physical facilities allow for flexibility in teaching methods, learning styles, and program scheduling	3.12	.87	2.90	.97	3.23	.84	3.24	.88	3.33	.77	4	2.61
(61) Physical facilities are accessible to providers	3.31	.82	3.09	.87	3.45	.70	3.41	.78	3.46	.72	4	3.93
(62) Physical facilities are accessible to participants	3.26	.85	3.10	.88	3.46	.71	3.42	.77	3.44	.71	4	3.96
(65) Storage space is accessible for material resources and educational records	3.10	.94	2.87	.96	3.27	.87	3.18	.94	3.27	.78	4	3.37
(80) Direct observations of critical care practice	3.32	.74	3.52	.57	3.62	.57	3.49	.71	3.49	.70	4	3.46
(96) Instructional objectives include application of knowledge and/or skills	3.44	.68	3.53	.59	3.54	.60	3.65	.56	3.35	.75	4	3.41

*All significant at P ≤ .01
Usefulness rating scale:
0 = Does not apply   2 = Moderately useful   4 = Extremely useful
1 = Not useful   3 = Quite useful

Table 22 shows that more experienced respondents (11+ years) view providers as more frequently assessing the validity and reliability of methods used for collection of assessment data prior to data analysis (72) than do less experienced educators (<2-3 years). When asked to judge the usefulness of program characteristics seven significant differences were identified. Table 23 presents the summary statistics from these comparisons.

There were five characteristics related to environmental resources that were found to be rated differently by respondents with varying levels of critical care education experience. When asked to judge the usefulness of physical facilities in attaining program goals (59), flexibility in arrangements (60) and accessibility to providers (61) and participants (62), the more experienced respondents (11+ years) rated these as more useful than did those less experienced (2-3 years). When asked to rate the usefulness of accessible storage space (65), the more experienced (4-5 and 11+ years) respondents saw it as more useful than those with less experience (2-3 years).

Respondents with different levels of critical care education experience differed significantly in their judgments of the usefulness of direct observation of critical care practice (80). Respondents in the 4-5 years of experience category differ significantly from those in the fewer than two years category. The higher experience category rated direct observation as more important than did the less experienced.

The remaining characteristic determined to differ significantly across levels of respondent experience in critical care education focused on the judged usefulness of whether instructional objectives include application of knowledge and/or skills (96). The more experienced group (11+ years) rated this characteristic lower than did the 6-10 years of experience group.

Respondents' area of practice. As shown in the table headings, area of practice was broken down into administration (director of critical care nursing, head nurse and supervisor), education (director of critical care education and critical care instructor), clinical (staff nurse and clinical nurse specialist) and private providers (continuing education providers). These categories are not to be confused with the three original categories used to identify critical care nursing educators to be surveyed. The comparison of mean ratings of frequency of occurrence of program characteristics by administrators, educators, clinicians and private providers of critical care educational service resulted in forty-one (N = 41) statistically significant results. Table 24 provides a summary of these significant F-tests.

Three characteristics related to material resources for programs were rated significantly different by types of educators. On the consistency of material resources to instructional objectives (53), availability (55), and sufficiency of reference materials (57) for instructional providers, educators consistently rated their frequency of occurrence higher than did administrators. This same relationship was true for frequency of occurrence of critical care supervisors assisting learners in identifying needs (68) and providers collaborating during assessment processes (75). Educators saw these program characteristics occurring more frequently than did the administrators.

With regard to data-gathering characteristics, private providers rated surveys, reports, questionnaires, market response (79) and prior program evaluations (86) as having a higher frequency of occurrence than the administrators. The frequency of

Table 24 ___ Summary of significant differences across areas of practice for frequency of occurrence of program characteristics

Program characteristics	Admin N = 296		Educ N = 262		Clin N = 75		Prvt N = 9		DF	F*
	X	SD	X	SD	X	SD	X	SD		
Material resources										
(53) Material resources used in critical care nursing education programs are consistent with the instructional objectives	4.03	.72	4.20	.67	3.95	.63	4.44	.52	3	4.73
(55) Up-to-date reference materials are available to providers	3.94	.84	4.21	.80	4.01	.91	4.25	1.03	3	4.76
(57) Sufficient reference materials are available to providers	3.81	.97	4.08	.89	3.93	.85	4.25	.70	3	4.08
Assessment of learning needs										
(68) Critical care supervisors assist learners in identifying individual and collective learning needs	3.87	.76	3.42	.93	3.64	.88	3.57	.78	3	12.10
(75) Prior to program planning, providers collaborate with critical care practitioners, supervisors, administrators and instructors to validate conclusions drawn during the assessment process	3.38	1.06	3.69	1.00	3.55	1.05	2.85	.89	3	4.52
Data gathering										
(79) Surveys, reports, questionnaires, marketing response	2.88	1.01	3.18	.84	3.02	.94	3.87	.83	3	6.33
(81) Results of quality assurance activities	3.67	.84	3.53	.87	3.45	.93	2.40	.89	3	4.73
(86) Prior program evaluations	3.44	1.02	3.82	.89	3.83	1.00	4.44	.72	3	9.54
Resources to achieve program goals										
(91) Environmental resources	3.08	1.03	3.38	1.04	3.14	1.08	3.11	1.05	3	3.82
Program goals and objectives										
(93) Program goals reflect the established priority of learning needs identified during the assessment process	3.79	.78	4.08	.67	3.95	.64	4.12	.64	3	6.95
(94) Instructional objectives are consistent with and further define the program goals	3.87	.83	4.39	.64	4.21	.72	4.33	.70	3	21.55
(95) Instructional objectives identify the cognitive, psychomotor, and/or affective behavior the learner will demonstrate following program participation	3.76	1.00	4.24	.88	4.29	.81	4.33	.70	3	13.55
(96) Instructional objectives include application of knowledge and/or skills	3.97	.80	4.24	.76	4.19	.74	4.00	1.22	3	5.50

*All significant at P ≤ .01

Frequency rating scale:

1 = Never	3 = Sometimes	5 = Always
2 = Seldom	4 = Frequently	

Table 24 —— Summary of significant differences across areas of practice for frequency of occurrence of program characteristics—cont'd

Program characteristics	Admin N = 296		Educ N = 262		Clin N = 75		Prvt N = 9		DF	F*
	X	SD	X	SD	X	SD	X	SD		
(97) Instructional objectives include clearly stated and measurable performance expectations of learners	3.89	.87	4.34	.73	4.21	.80	4.33	1.00	3	11.69
(98) Content of the curriculum is selected and leveled to facilitate learner attainment of the instructional objectives	3.89	.81	4.32	.64	4.26	.65	4.66	.50	3	17.82
(99) The sequencing of learning experiences considers the content to be presented and characteristics of the learner (educational and experiential background)	3.77	.87	4.13	.73	4.01	.76	3.75	1.03	3	8.9
(100) Instructional hours are allocated on the basis of instructional objectives, complexity of the content, level of instruction, and resource availability	3.76	1.03	4.12	.78	4.10	.85	3.88	1.26	3	7.13
(101) Providers select instructional media that are current, accurate, and consistent with the instructional objectives	4.02	.75	4.29	.62	4.14	.63	4.22	.66	3	6.56
Program formats										
(102) Size of the learner group	4.00	.90	4.25	.77	4.15	.71	4.62	.51	3	5.11
(103) Breadth of content to be addressed	4.10	.83	4.39	.62	4.26	.60	4.37	.51	3	7.05
(104) Level of instruction (beginning, intermediate, or advanced)	4.14	.82	4.39	.68	4.28	.66	4.22	.44	3	4.77
(105) Application of principles of adult education	3.83	.93	4.29	.76	4.21	.67	4.22	.66	3	13.61
Evaluation strategy										
(110) Providers develop a strategy to evaluate application of learning to critical care nursing practice	3.38	1.04	3.68	1.03	3.54	.95	2.85	1.34	3	4.66
(111) Providers select and/or design tools for evaluating the program and learning	3.52	1.10	4.12	.94	4.01	.87	4.44	.52	3	17.27
(112) Providers select and validate tools which contain the criteria to be used during the evaluation process	3.29	1.10	3.65	1.11	3.36	1.01	3.62	1.18	3	4.75
Program implementation										
(114) Providers delineate prerequisite/entry requirements for each offering within the educational program	3.28	1.13	3.63	1.11	3.64	.98	3.33	1.22	3	4.55
(116) Providers establish a time schedule of offerings in the educational program	3.93	1.02	4.35	.78	4.31	.84	4.33	1.11	3	10.14

Continued.

Table 24 —— Summary of significant differences across areas of practice for frequency of occurrence of program characteristics—cont'd

Program characteristics	Admin N = 296		Educ N = 262		Clin N = 75		Prvt N = 9		DF	F*
	X	SD	X	SD	X	SD	X	SD		
Program implementation — cont'd										
(117) Program implementation is consistent with the instructional objectives, curriculum and format selected for the program	3.92	.85	4.37	.65	4.23	.64	4.33	.70	3	16.44
(118) Program implementation is consistent with the plan for program initiation and the established administrative framework for critical care educational programs	3.75	.90	4.10	.76	9.02	.76	4.00	.81	3	7.65
(120) Providers modify the program based upon discrepancies between planned and actual implementation	3.53	.97	3.91	.90	3.66	.79	4.00	1.32	3	7.37
(121) Providers afford learners opportunities for active participation in the learning experience	4.02	.81	4.24	.63	4.05	.70	4.11	.78	3	4.30
(122) Providers incorporate the learner's life and work experience in instructional activities	3.65	.93	3.91	.80	3.69	.84	4.11	1.05	3	4.56
(123) Providers offer learners immediate feedback and reinforcement of learning	3.79	.89	4.08	.69	3.94	.77	4.11	.92	3	5.81
(125) Instructors interact with learners in a constructive and supportive manner	4.15	.77	4.41	.55	4.31	.54	4.55	.72	3	7.23
(126) Instructors establish a climate of openness and mutual respect in their interactions with learners	4.19	.78	4.48	.56	4.39	.56	4.55	.72	3	8.38
Program evaluation										
(136) Critical care instructors participate in program evaluation	3.95	1.00	4.38	.81	4.39	.72	4.12	.64	3	8.27
(139) Providers evaluate program effectiveness in meeting learning needs of the critical care nurse	3.85	.89	4.12	.82	3.94	.87	4.22	.66	3	4.33
(141) Providers evaluate programs relative to the realities of the critical care practice setting	3.84	.88	4.09	.76	3.95	.74	4.12	.64	3	3.89
(143) Providers evaluate programs relative to the standards of applicable professional accrediting bodies and/or regulatory agencies	3.68	.97	3.96	.94	3.93	.83	4.37	.74	3	4.82
(152) Providers evaluate the program relative to learner's attainment of instructional objectives	3.71	.95	4.00	.79	4.02	.77	4.00	.63	3	5.65
(155) Providers periodically revise programs based on the data contained in the evaluative records	3.79	.92	4.19	.72	4.13	.85	4.50	.53	3	11.39

program evaluations was rated significantly lower by administrators when compared to educators, clinicians and private providers. The results of quality assurance activities (81) was rated lower on frequency of occurrence by private providers when compared to both administrators and educators.

Only one of five statements related to resources to achieve program goals was found to differ in rated frequency of occurrence across areas of practice. Educators rated the frequency with which environmental resources are analyzed to determine compatibility with program goals (91) as significantly higher than did administrators.

Each of the nine program characteristics presented under the heading of program goals and objectives was rated by administrators as having a lower frequency of occurrence when compared to educators' responses (93-101). Clinicians also differed significantly from administrators on four characteristics (94, 95, 97, 98). Like the educators, clinicians rated the frequency of occurrence of these characteristics higher than did the administrators. Private providers rated highest the frequency with which the content of the curriculum is selected and leveled to facilitate learner attainment of the instructional objectives (98). Private providers differed significantly in their ratings compared to administrators.

Educators again rated consideration of size of learner group (102), breadth of content to be addressed (103), level of instruction (104) and the application of principles of adult education (105) as more frequently occurring than did administrators. Clinicians also differed significantly from administrators on the application of principles of adult education.

Table 24 also presents the comparison of the three significant program characteristics grouped under the heading of evaluation strategy (110, 111, 112). Administrators rated the frequency of occurrence of these items lower than did the educators. Clinicians had a slightly lower average rating than the educators but their responses differed significantly from those of the administrators.

Ten of the fourteen characteristics labeled as program implementation were rated as differing by categories of area of practice. Educators consistently rated these frequencies higher than did administrators. In two instances (116, 117) the clinicians also differed significantly from the administrators. No other paired comparisons were found to be significant.

Of the fourteen statements that comprised the program evaluation grouping of characteristics, six were found to have ratings that differ significantly across areas of practice. Again, educators rated the frequency of occurrence of critical care instructors participating in program evaluations (136), providers evaluating program effectiveness in terms of meeting learning needs (139), being consistent with realities of the critical care practice setting (141), and meeting applicable professional accrediting bodies' standards (143) and relationship to learners' attainment of instructional objectives (152) significantly higher than did administrators. Educators also rated the frequency with which programs are revised based on evaluative records (152) significantly higher than did the administrators.

Comparisons across areas of practice were also performed on respondent ratings of usefulness of program characteristics. Eighteen comparisons across categories of areas of practice found to have significant mean differences on ratings of usefulness are presented in Table 25.

Table 25 ── Summary of significant differences across areas of practice for usefulness of program characteristics

Program characteristics	Admin N = 286		Educ N = 262		Clin N = 75		Prvt N = 9		DF	F*
	X	SD	X	SD	X	SD	X	SD		
Program elements										
(7) Periodic performance appraisals for those providing critical care nursing	3.36	.75	3.05	.93	3.27	.85	3.00	1.00	3	5.84
(13) Documentation of actual revenue and expenses	2.96	.91	2.71	.86	2.76	.83	3.87	.35	3	6.18
Material resources										
(55) Up-to-date reference materials are available to providers	3.43	.73	3.62	.62	3.65	.63	3.62	.74	3	4.49
Environmental resources										
(66) Clinical experiences are available to meet the instructional objectives related to nursing practice	3.34	.78	3.57	.63	3.62	.69	3.50	.57	3	5.68
Data gathering										
(86) Prior program evaluations	3.00	.88	3.12	.78	3.41	.82	3.88	.33	3	7.19
Program goals and objectives										
(94) Instructional objectives are consistent with and further define the program goals	3.26	.76	3.58	.57	3.49	.55	3.55	.72	3	9.92
(95) Instructional objectives identify the cognitive, psychomotor, and/or affective behavior the learner will demonstrate following program participation	3.25	.77	3.51	.64	3.57	.55	3.44	1.01	3	6.91
(97) Instructional objectives include clearly stated and measurable performance expectations of learners	3.41	.68	3.60	.60	3.54	.58	3.22	1.09	3	4.42
(98) Content of the curriculum is selected and leveled to facilitate learner attainment of the instructional objectives	3.37	.69	3.57	.60	3.58	.55	3.88	.33	3	5.69
(99) The sequencing of learning experiences considers the content to be presented and characteristics of the learner (educational and experiential background)	3.28	.73	3.51	.62	3.45	.65	3.50	.75	3	4.90
Program formats										
(105) Application of principles of adult education	3.31	.72	3.55	.58	3.52	.60	3.66	.50	3	6.37

*All significant at P ≤ .01
Usefulness scale:
1 = Not useful   3 = Quite useful
2 = Moderately useful   4 = Extremely useful

Table 25 —— Summary of significant differences across areas of practice for usefulness of program characteristics—cont'd

Program characteristics	Admin N = 286		Educ N = 262		Clin N = 75		Prvt N = 9		DF	F*
	X	SD	X	SD	X	SD	X	SD		
Evaluation strategy										
(109) Both program evaluation and evaluation of learning are included in the evaluation process	3.37	.70	3.54	.66	3.67	.58	3.66	.50	3	4.91
(110) Providers develop a strategy to evaluate application of learning to critical care nursing practice	3.20	.79	3.42	.73	3.52	.69	3.00	1.15	3	5.14
(111) Providers select and/or design tools for evaluating the program and learning	3.24	.75	3.46	.69	3.47	.71	3.44	.72	3	4.25
Program implementation										
(117) Program implementation is consistent with the instructional objectives, curriculum and format selected for the program	3.37	.71	3.61	.54	3.57	.64	3.77	.44	3	6.72
(123) Providers offer learners immediate feedback and reinforcement of learning	3.46	.68	3.65	.54	3.64	.58	3.66	.70	3	4.29
(126) Instructors establish a climate of openness and mutual respect in their interactions with learners	3.67	.55	3.81	.40	3.82	.38	3.88	.33	3	4.57
Program evaluation										
(136) Critical care instructors participate in program evaluation	3.44	.67	3.63	.54	3.66	.53	3.37	.74	3	4.81

With regard to the usefulness of periodic appraisals of those providing critical care nursing (7), administrators rated this item significantly higher than did educators. Clinicians had the next highest rating but this mean value did not differ significantly from any other category of respondent. The second program element whose ratings of usefulness differed across groups related to the documentation of actual revenue and expenses (13). Private providers differed significantly from all other categories of area of practice with the highest mean rating of usefulness. The educators had the lowest rating of usefulness.

Having up-to-date reference materials available (55) was rated significantly more useful by educators than by administrators. The educators also rated higher the usefulness of having clinical experiences available to meet the instructional objectives (66) than did the administrators. The highest rating of usefulness on this characteristic (66) was made by clinicians, who also differed significantly from administrators. The usefulness of one data-gathering device (prior program evaluations, #86) was found to differ significantly among groups of respondents. Specifically, private providers and clinicians differed significantly from the administrators on the ratings of usefulness. Clinicians and private providers rated the usefulness of prior program evaluations higher than did administrators.

Five of the nine characteristics related to program goals and objectives were found to have usefulness ratings that differed significantly across areas of practice (94, 95, 97, 98, 99). Educators consistently rated the usefulness of each characteristic higher than did administrators. Clinicians significantly rated higher than administrators the usefulness of instructional objectives which identify the cognitive, psychomotor, and/or affective behavior the learner will demonstrate following program participation (95).

When asked to rate the usefulness of the application of principles of adult education (105), educators rated this program characteristic as significantly more useful than did administrators. Even though private providers (N = 9) rated this program characteristic the highest of all groups, the post-hoc analysis did not show a significant difference between private providers and any other group.

Educators and administrators again differed significantly in terms of their ratings of usefulness of evaluation strategies. Educators rated the inclusion of both program and learning evaluation in programs (109), the evaluation of the application of learning to critical care nursing practice (110) as well as the selection and/or design of evaluation tools (111) as more useful than did administrators. Program characteristics 109 and 110 were rated by clinicians as the most useful, differing significantly from the administrators.

Three program characteristics related to program implementation were found to have ratings of usefulness that differ significantly across areas of practice. The implementation of the program consistent with its instructional objectives (117), the provision of immediate feedback to learners (123) and the establishment by instructors of a climate of openness and mutual respect (126) were all rated as more useful by educators than by administrators. Private providers had the highest ratings but they did not differ significantly from any of the other groups.

When asked to rate the usefulness of critical care instructors participating in program evaluations (136), educators rated this involvement as more useful than did the administrators.

Respondents were asked to indicate the frequency with which stated program characteristics were evaluated by providers and learners of critical care education. Table 26 provides the significant comparisons across groups within area of practice.

Educators consistently rated providers as more frequently performing the following items when compared to administrators:

    a. Relevance and priority of instructional objectives (IO) (144)
    b. Behavioral and measurable attributes of IO (145)
    c. Consistency and correlation between IO and instructional content (146)
    d. Effectiveness of instructors (148)
    e. Quality of instruction (149)
    f. Impact of learning environment in facilitating learning (150).

Table 26 ___ Summary of significant differences across areas of practice for frequency of evaluation by providers

Program characteristics	Admin N = 286		Educ N = 262		Clin N = 75		Prvt N = 9		DF	F*
	X	SD	X	SD	X	SD	X	SD		
(144) Relevance and priority of instructional objectives (IO)	3.76	.91	4.15	.83	4.05	.80	4.12	.83	3	8.77
(145) Behavioral and measurable attributes of IO	3.59	1.00	4.02	.86	3.95	.95	4.42	.78	3	10.42
(146) Consistency and correlation between IO and instructional content	3.71	.99	4.20	.85	4.06	.81	4.85	.37	3	14.66
(148) Effectiveness of instructors	3.81	.95	4.25	.86	4.21	.86	4.50	.75	3	11.51
(149) Quality of instruction	3.86	.92	4.31	.80	4.18	.83	4.62	.51	3	12.91
(150) Impact of learning environment in facilitating learning	3.63	1.05	4.05	.93	3.85	.96	4.12	.64	3	7.91

*All significant at $P \leq .01$
0 = Not applicable   2 = Seldom   4 = Frequently
1 = Never   3 = Sometimes   5 = Always

Clinicians also rated providers as more frequently performing 145, 146, 148, 149 than did administrators. The highest rating of the frequency with which providers assured the consistency, validity and correlation between instructional objectives and evaluation tools used to validate learning acquisition (146) was given by private providers. This rating also differed significantly from that given by administrators but did not differ from any other group.

The same program characteristics were also rated in terms of the frequency with which they are evaluated by learners. Three significant differences were found across areas of practice and are presented in Table 27.

Educators rated the frequency with which learners evaluate the effectiveness of instructors (148), the quality of instruction (149) and the impact of learning environment in facilitating learning (150) higher than did administrators. No other differences were found between groups of respondents.

Table 28 presents a summary of the significant differences across area of practice on selected program characteristics that fall under the heading of human resources.

When asked to indicate the percentage of instructors meeting the nursing practice standards of the critical care unit in their area of teaching assignment (36), the responses of educators and clinicians differed significantly from those of administrators. Clinicians indicated that ninety-five percent (95.39%) and educators indicated ninety-three percent (92.69%) of the instructors meet the standards. Administrators indicated that seventy-nine percent (79.45%) meet the practice standards. The small group of private providers indicated that only fifty-five percent (55%) meet the standards.

Table 27 ___ Summary of significant differences across areas of practice for frequency of evaluation by learners

Program characteristics	Admin N = 286		Educ N = 262		Clin N = 75		Prvt N = 9		DF	F*
	X	SD	X	SD	X	SD	X	SD		
(148) Effectiveness of instructors	3.94	.91	4.28	.80	4.15	.82	4.75	.46	3	8.17
(149) Quality of instruction	3.91	.95	4.28	.77	4.15	.83	4.75	.46	3	9.40
(150) Impact of learning environment in facilitating learning	3.56	1.10	3.88	.98	3.77	1.02	3.87	1.35	3	3.88

*All significant at P ≤ .01

0 = Not applicable	2 = Seldom	4 = Frequently
1 = Never	3 = Sometimes	5 = Always

Table 28 ___ Summary of significant differences across areas of practice on selected human resources program characteristics

Program characteristics	Admin N = 286		Educ N = 262		Clin N = 75		Prvt N = 9		DF	F*
	X	SD	X	SD	X	SD	X	SD		
(36) What percent of instructors meet the nursing practice standards of the critical care unit in their area of teaching assignment?	79.45	35.42	92.69	22.39	95.39	15.41	55.00	63.63	3	9.46
(37) What percent of instructors demonstrate competence in the application of nursing and scientific concepts and principles of care of the critically ill patient?	86.69	28.99	93.43	21.29	96.80	13.67	80.00	28.28	3	3.87
(38) Are the existing selection criteria for critical care nursing instructors consistent with program goals?	2.52	.95	2.95	.87	2.95	.79	3.75	.50	3	11.01

*All significant at P ≤ .01

Scale values:

1 = Not very much	3 = Quite
2 = Moderately	4 = Extremely

The respondents were somewhat more congruent in their indication of the percent of instructors who demonstrate competence in the application of nursing and scientific concepts and principles to the care of the critically ill patient (37). Clinicians indicated that ninety-seven percent (96.80%) meet the level of competency, which was significantly different from administrators (86.69%). The private providers rated the level of competence lowest (80%).

Program characteristic #38 asked the survey respondents to indicate the degree to which the existing selection criteria for critical care nursing instructors are consistent with program goals. On a four-point scale (1 = not very much, 2 = moderately, 3 = quite, 4 = extremely), clinicians and educators differed from administrators in their ratings. Educators and clinicians rated this characteristic significantly higher than did administrators.

Respondents' location. The following information is a presentation of the results of comparing respondents' ratings of the program characteristics by whether they are from rural, suburban or urban practice settings.

Table 29 presents the means and standard deviations for each of the categories of location along with the degrees of freedom and associated F-values.

Two program characteristics classified as material resources were found to have significantly different ratings by respondents' location. Respondents from urban and suburban locations rated availability of sufficient reference materials for providers (57) and participants (58) as significantly higher than did those from rural locations. The suburban and urban respondents also rated clinical experiences as more frequently available to meet the instructional objectives related to nursing practice (66) than did rural respondents. The frequency with which providers assess the validity and reliability of methods used for collection of assessment data prior to data analysis (72) was rated higher by those from suburban locations than by those from rural or urban locations.

Of the eight significant mean score comparisons across locations for the one data-gathering characteristic (79), the four goals and objectives (93, 94, 95, 97) and three program implementation characteristics, respondents from rural locations rated their frequency of occurrence significantly lower than did the suburban and urban respondents. The only exception was a nonsignificant post-hoc comparison between rural and suburban respondents on instructional objectives being clearly stated as measurable expectations of learners (97).

When asked about the participation of critical care instructors in program evaluations (136), urban respondents had the highest mean rating and differed significantly from the suburban as well as the rural respondents. The suburban and urban respondents more frequently incorporate formative and summative evaluations into programs (154) and revise programs based on the data contained in the evaluative records (155) than do rural respondents.

The ratings of usefulness of program characteristics by respondents from categories of location are presented in Table 30.

Table 29 — Summary of significant differences across locations for frequency of occurrence of program characteristics

Program characteristics	Rural N = 150 X	Rural N = 150 SD	Suburban N = 156 X	Suburban N = 156 SD	Urban N = 195 X	Urban N = 195 SD	DF	F*
Material resources								
(57) Sufficient reference materials are available to providers	3.69	1.01	4.07	.92	3.95	.88		6.21
(58) Sufficient reference materials are available to participants	3.67	.98	4.04	.91	3.85	.92	2	5.68
Environmental resources								
(66) Clinical experiences are available to meet the instructional objectives related to nursing practice	3.50	.90	3.76	.88	3.79	.82	2	5.13
Assessment of learning needs								
(72) Providers assess the validity and reliability of methods used for collection of assessment data prior to data analysis	2.90	1.07	3.33	1.09	2.89	1.11	2	7.38
Data gathering								
(79) Surveys, reports, questionnaires, marketing response	2.80	.97	3.21	.96	3.07	90	2	6.45
Program goals and objectives								
(93) Program goals reflect the established priority of learning needs identified during the assessment process	3.79	.71	4.02	.74	4.03	.69	2	5.03
(94) Instructional objectives are consistent with and further define the program goals	3.93	.81	4.23	.74	4.29	.65	2	10.09
(95) Instructional objectives identify the cognitive, psychomotor, and/or affective behavior the learner will demonstrate following program participation	3.78	1.04	4.15	.90	4.16	.90	2	7.27
(97) Instructional objectives include clearly stated and measurable performance expectations of learners	3.95	.87	4.19	.82	4.23	.74	2	5.21
Program implementation								
(113) Providers establish maximum and minimum enrollments for each offering in the educational program	3.20	1.24	3.73	1.12	3.59	1.13	2	10.34
(117) Program implementation is consistent with the instructional objectives, curriculum and format selected for the program	3.93	.86	4.23	.75	4.30	.66	2	5.77
(120) Providers modify the program based upon discrepancies between planned and actual implementation	3.49	.99	3.77	.96	3.83	.84	2	5.43
Program evaluation								
(136) Critical care instructors participate in program evaluation	4.00	.98	4.12	.97	4.36	.83	2	6.25
(154) Providers incorporate both formative and summative evaluations of the program	3.13	1.14	3.46	1.18	3.51	1.06	2	4.70
(155) Providers periodically revise programs based on the data contained in the evaluative records	3.78	.86	4.01	.92	4.17	.76	2	5.99

*All significant at $P \leq .01$

Frequency rating scale
0 = Does not apply   2 = Seldom   4 = Frequently
1 = Never   3 = Sometimes   5 = Always

Table 30 ___ Summary of significant differences across locations for usefulness of program characteristics

Program characteristics	Rural N = 150		Suburban N = 156		Urban N = 195		DF	F*
	X	SD	X	SD	X	SD		
Program elements								
(15) Documentation of program evaluation	3.09	.79	3.36	.73	3.36	.74	2	5.46
Material resources								
(53) Material resources used in critical care nursing education programs are consistent with the instructional objectives	3.21	.78	3.45	.64	3.47	.62	2	6.41
(54) Instructional aids are accurate and current	3.30	.80	3.54	.66	3.53	.65	2	5.25
(58) Sufficient reference materials are available to participants	3.30	.82	3.49	.71	3.55	.66	2	5.03
Environmental resources								
(64) Storage space is available for material resources and educational records	2.97	.98	3.08	.91	3.28	.81	2	5.08
(66) Clinical experiences are available to meet the instructional objectives related to nursing practice	3.36	.77	3.45	.71	3.63	.64	2	6.04
Assessment of learning needs								
(67) Learners have primary responsibility for the identification of their own learning needs	3.10	.87	3.26	.77	3.39	.70	2	3.35
(72) Providers assess the validity and reliability of methods used for collection of assessment data prior to data analysis	2.69	.96	3.02	.87	3.03	.91	2	5.55
(73) Providers analyze trends in assessment information	2.64	1.00	3.00	.92	3.09	.85	2	8.11
Program goals and objectives								
(93) Program goals reflect the established priority of learning needs identified during the assessment process	3.24	.71	3.41	.62	3.46	.60	2	4.99
(94) Instructional objectives are consistent with and further define the program goals	3.24	.79	3.48	.60	3.60	.54	2	11.96
(95) Instructional objectives identify the cognitive, psychomotor, and/or affective behavior the learner will demonstrate following program participation	3.21	.80	3.45	.63	3.52	.64	2	8.45
(96) Instructional objectives include application of knowledge and/or skills	3.42	.64	3.54	.58	3.64	.54	2	5.07
(97) Instructional objectives include clearly stated and measurable performance expectations of learners	3.39	.66	3.53	.64	3.63	.55	2	5.88
(98) Content of the curriculum is selected and leveled to facilitate learner attainment of the instructional objectives	3.35	.68	3.54	.64	3.58	.56	2	5.29
(99) The sequencing of learning experiences considers the content to be presented and characteristics of the learner (educational and experiential background)	3.27	.69	3.43	.69	3.53	.60	2	5.90

*All are significant at $P \leq .01$
1 = Not useful   3 = Quite useful
2 = Moderately useful   4 = Extremely useful   *Continued.*

Table 30 —— Summary of significant differences across locations for usefulness of program characteristics —cont'd

Program characteristics	Rural N = 150		Suburban N = 156		Urban N = 195		DF	F*
	X	SD	X	SD	X	SD		
Program format								
(106) Amount of time available for preparation and implementation of the program	3.30	.75	3.49	.65	3.57	.65	2	6.09
(110) Providers develop a strategy to evaluate application of learning to critical care nursing practice	3.13	.82	3.34	.77	3.50	.69	2	5.07
(111) Providers select and/or design tools for evaluating the program and learning	3.14	.76	3.40	.73	3.55	.60	2	13.32
(112) Providers select and validate tools which contain the criteria to be used during the evaluation process	2.99	.83	3.30	.78	3.37	.72	2	5.73
Program implementation								
(116) Providers establish a time schedule of offerings in the educational program	3.31	.74	3.50	.67	3.56	.59	2	5.49
(117) Program implementation is consistent with the instructional objectives, curriculum and format selected for the program	3.30	.74	3.55	.60	3.62	.55	2	4.10
(118) Program implementation is consistent with the plan for program initiation and the established administrative framework for critical care educational programs	3.17	.76	3.35	.68	3.53	.58	2	10.19
Program evaluation								
(136) Critical care instructors participate in program evaluation	3.37	.69	3.56	.64	3.65	.51	2	7.70
(139) Providers evaluate program effectiveness in meeting learning needs of the critical care nurse	3.30	.74	3.53	.61	3.59	.61	2	7.90
(141) Providers evaluate programs relative to the realities of the critical care practice setting	3.36	.74	3.51	.63	3.61	.56	2	5.87
(151) Providers evaluate the program relative to learners' ability to apply learning in critical care nursing practice	3.16	.75	3.43	.69	3.55	.62	2	12.47
(152) Providers evaluate the program relative to learners' attainment of instructional objectives	3.26	.75	3.43	.67	3.51	.58	2	2.34
(153) Providers evaluate the program relative to the adequacy of resources needed to support the program	3.01	.84	3.21	.82	3.30	.78	2	4.70
(154) Providers incorporate both formative and summative evaluations of the program	2.87	.93	3.16	.80	3.25	.77	2	5.25
(155) Providers periodically revise programs based on the data contained in the evaluative records	3.41	.69	3.59	.54	3.70	.51	2	9.13

In all cases the mean rating of usefulness for the urban respondents on each characteristic was significantly higher than the mean for the rural respondents. The mean ratings of the suburban respondents were all higher than those of the rural respondents but only nineteen of the thirty-two relationships presented demonstrated statistically significant post-hoc comparisons between suburban and rural respondents. When asked to rate the usefulness of having program implementations consistent with the plan for program initiation and established administrative frameworks for critical care educational programs (118), the urban and suburban respondents differed significantly from each other. The urban respondents rated this characteristic as significantly more useful than did the suburban respondents. This was the only significant difference between the urban and suburban respondents.

The frequency with which program characteristics are evaluated by providers and learners was rated by respondents. Table 31 presents the results of the comparison of respondents from the three categories of location on the frequency of evaluations by providers.

The relevance and priority of instructional objectives (144), the behavioral and measurable attributes of instructional objectives (145), the effectiveness of instructors (148) and the quality of instruction (149) were all rated as occurring more frequently by the urban respondents than by rural respondents. The mean ratings of the suburban and urban respondents do not differ significantly from each other.

Table 32 presents the ratings by location of the frequency with which program characteristics are evaluated by learners.

The evaluation of instructor effectiveness (148) and the impact of the learning environment in facilitating learning (150) were rated as occurring significantly more frequently by the urban respondents in comparison to rural respondents. Likewise, the suburban respondents rated the frequency of evaluation of instructor effectiveness and the impact of the learning environment significantly higher than did the rural respondents. The urban respondents rated the evaluation of the quality of instruction as occurring more frequently than the rural respondents. Even though the mean of the suburban respondents was higher than that of the rural respondents, no significant post-hoc comparison was found.

The comparison of the percentage of instructors who meet the nursing practice standards of the critical care unit in their area of teaching assignment (36) by location is presented in Table 33.

A significant difference exists between the judgments of urban respondents and rural respondents. The urban respondents indicate that ninety-two percent (91.72%) meet this standard while the rural respondents report that seventy-nine percent (78.52%) meet this requirement. The suburban respondents (89.10%) did not differ significantly from either the rural or urban respondents.

Respondents' experience in critical care nursing. Comparisons of ratings of program characteristics were analyzed by five categories of years of critical care nursing experience (<4, 4-5, 6-10, 11-15, 16+). The following tables present the results of significant F-tests comparing ratings of frequency of occurrence and usefulness ratings of program characteristics.

Table 31 ___ Summary of significant differences across locations for frequency of evaluations by providers

Program characteristics	Rural N = 150		Suburban N = 156		Urban N = 195		DF	F*
	X	SD	X	SD	X	SD		
(144) Relevance and priority of instructional objectives (IO)	3.77	.94	4.04	.88	4.03	.86	2	5.09
(145) Behavioral and measurable attributes of IO	3.61	.98	3.92	.98	3.92	.93	2	5.02
(148) Effectiveness of instructors	3.80	1.02	4.00	1.02	4.22	.83	2	7.79
(149) Quality of instruction	3.87	.93	4.06	.97	4.25	.81	2	5.66

*All significant at P ≤ .01
Frequency rating scale:
0 = Not applicable   2 = Seldom   4 = Frequently
1 = Never   3 = Sometimes   5 = Always

Table 32 ___ Summary of significant differences across locations for frequency of evaluations by learners

Program characteristics	Rural N = 150		Suburban N = 156		Urban N = 195		DF	F*
	X	SD	X	SD	X	SD		
(148) Effectiveness of instructors	3.85	.94	4.14	.90	4.28	.80	2	9.02
(149) Quality of instruction	3.91	.88	4.10	.91	4.26	.84	2	6.05
(150) Impact of learning environment in facilitating learning	3.50	1.07	3.77	1.11	3.88	.99	2	5.08

*All significant at P ≤ .01
Frequency rating scale:
0 = Not applicable   2 = Seldom   4 = Frequently
1 = Never   3 = Sometimes   5 = Always

Table 33 ___ Summary of significant differences across locations on the percentage of critical care instructors meeting practice standards

Program characteristics	Rural N = 150		Suburban N = 156		Urban N = 195		DF	F*
	X	SD	X	SD	X	SD		
(36) What percent of instructors meet the nursing practice standards of the critical care unit in their area of teaching assignment?	78.52	36.10	89.10	27.84	91.72	22.65	2	7.51

*All significant at P ≤ .01

Table 34 —— Summary of significant differences across categories of years of critical care nursing experience for frequency of occurrence of program characteristics

Program characteristics	<4 N = 37		4-5 N = 87		6-10 N = 241		11-15 N = 191		16+ N = 75		DF	F*
	X	SD	X	SD	X	SD	X	SD	X	SD		
(58) Sufficient reference materials are available to participants	3.61	1.10	3.78	.79	3.93	.94	3.85	.94	4.20	.90	4	3.34
(116) Providers establish a time schedule of offerings in the educational program	3.64	1.06	4.06	.97	4.27	.82	4.15	.94	4.31	.93	4	4.28

*All significant at $P \leq .01$
Frequency rating scale:
0 = Does not apply	2 = Seldom	4 = Frequently
1 = Never	3 = Sometimes	5 = Always

Table 34 presents two program characteristics for which there is a significant difference across categories of experience in critical care nursing.

Those respondents with fewer than four years of critical care nursing experience rated the frequency of having sufficient reference materials available to participants (58) and the scheduling of offerings in educational programs (116) significantly lower than did respondents with sixteen or more years of experience. The fewer than four years of experience group was also significantly lower than the respondents from the six to ten years of experience group. No other program characteristic had significant differences in ratings across categories of critical care nursing experience.

When rated for usefulness by respondents with varying levels of experience, four program characteristics demonstrated significant differences in group means. Table 35 presents the results of these comparisons.

The usefulness of position descriptions for all involved in critical care nursing education (9) was rated by those with sixteen or more years of experience as more useful than by those with six to ten years of experience. No other categories of experience differed significantly on their ratings of usefulness with regard to program characteristic #9.

Respondents with fewer than four years of experience rated the usefulness of the content of the curriculum selected and leveled to facilitate learner attainment of the instructional objectives (98) as significantly lower than did those with six to ten years of experience. No other comparisons on this program characteristic across levels of experience were significant even though the means of the eleven to fifteen and sixteen plus categories were close to the mean of the six to ten category of years of experience.

When rating the usefulness of providers establishing a time schedule of offerings in the educational program (116), respondents in the six to ten, eleven to fifteen and the sixteen plus years of experience categories were significantly higher than those in the fewer than four years of experience group of respondents. This same relationship was true for the usefulness of program implementation consistent with the instructional objectives, curriculum and format selected for the program (117). The ratings of usefulness by respondents from the four to five years of critical care nursing experience did not differ significantly from any other experience category.

Table 36 presents the means and standard deviations for the ratings of frequency of evaluation of learners on the effectiveness of instructors. Respondents with six to ten and eleven to fifteen years of nursing experience rated the frequency of occurrence of instructor effectiveness evaluations (148) higher than did those with fewer than four years of experience.

Table 35 ___ Summary of significant differences across categories of years of critical care nursing experience for usefulness of program characteristics

Program characteristics	<4 N = 37		4-5 N = 87		6-10 N = 241		11-15 N = 191		16+ N = 75		DF	F*
	X	SD	X	SD	X	SD	X	SD	X	SD		
(9) Position descriptions for all involved in critical care nursing education	3.00	.90	3.07	.98	2.75	.96	3.04	.92	3.22	.79	4	3.91
(98) Content of the curriculum is selected and leveled to facilitate learner attainment of the instructional objectives	3.14	.92	3.37	.68	3.57	.58	3.51	.62	3.50	.61	4	4.12
(116) Providers establish a time schedule of offerings in the educational program	3.03	.72	3.43	.68	3.49	.62	3.44	.71	3.53	.69	4	3.66
(117) Program implementation is consistent with the instructional objectives, curriculum and format selected for the program	3.14	.70	3.44	.66	3.51	.62	3.55	.62	3.60	.62	4	3.64

*All significant at P ≤ .01
Usefulness rating scale:
0 = Does not apply   2 = Moderately useful   4 = Extremely useful
1 = Not useful   3 = Quite useful

Table 36 ___ Summary of significant differences across categories of years of critical care nursing experience for frequency of evaluation by learners

Program characteristics	<4 N = 37		4-5 N = 87		6-10 N = 241		11-15 N = 191		16+ N = 75		DF	F*
	X	SD	X	SD	X	SD	X	SD	X	SD		
(148) Effectiveness of instructors	3.60	1.11	4.02	.91	4.19	.79	4.18	.82	4.11	.97	4	3.83

*All significant at P ≤ .01
Frequency rating scale:
0 = Not applicable   2 = Seldom   4 = Frequently
1 = Never   3 = Sometimes   5 = Always

Respondents' hospital size. A comparison was made of ratings of program characteristics by respondents from different sized hospitals. Ratings were made by respondents in terms of the frequency of occurrence and usefulness to programs of each program characteristic.

Table 37 presents the significant comparisons across categories of hospital size for twenty program characteristics.

Table 37 ——— Summary of significant differences across hospital size for frequency of occurrence of program characteristics

Program characteristics	<100 N = 70		100-199 N = 60		200-299 N = 74		300-399 N = 48		400+ N = 72		DF	F*
	X	SD	X	SD	X	SD	X	SD	X	SD		
Material resources												
(57) Sufficient reference materials are available to providers	3.61	.92	3.67	1.09	3.93	.93	3.84	.94	4.16	.89	4	4.26
Environmental resources												
(66) Clinical experiences are available to meet the instructional objectives related to nursing practice	3.43	.78	3.38	.97	3.91	.82	3.68	.86	3.88	.77	4	8.51
Assessment of learning needs												
(76) Providers establish priorities among learning needs relative to the philosophy and goals of the program and available resources	4.00	.71	3.60	.95	4.05	.75	4.15	.75	4.07	.76	4	4.21
Data gathering												
(86) Prior program evaluations	3.32	1.07	3.35	.97	3.64	.91	3.85	.77	3.79	.99	4	6.04
Program goals and objectives												
(93) Program goals reflect the established priority of learning needs identified during the assessment process	3.96	.55	3.61	.85	4.05	.69	4.10	.63	4.13	.72	4	6.08
(94) Instructional objectives are consistent with and further define the program goals	4.05	.70	3.85	.92	4.40	.62	4.31	.75	4.34	.66	4	7.30

*All significant at P ≤ .01
Frequency rating scale:
0 = Does not apply   2 = Seldom   4 = Frequently
1 = Never   3 = Sometimes   5 = Always   *Continued.*

Table 37 ___ Summary of significant differences across hospital size
for frequency of occurrence of program characteristics—cont'd

Program characteristics	<100 N = 70		100-199 N = 60		200-299 N = 74		300-399 N = 48		400+ N = 72		DF	F*
	X	SD	X	SD	X	SD	X	SD	X	SD		
Program goals and objectives — cont'd												
(95) Instructional objectives identify the cognitive, psychomotor, and/or affective behavior the learner will demonstrate following program participation	3.80	.90	3.76	1.11	4.15	.88	4.44	.74	4.31	.83	4	5.53
(97) Instructional objectives include clearly stated and measurable performance expectations of learners	4.01	.80	3.83	.94	4.23	.79	4.42	.68	4.30	.67	4	5.62
(98) Content of the curriculum is selected and leveled to facilitate learner attainment of the instructional objectives	4.06	.65	3.76	.91	4.26	.71	4.28	.68	4.31	.65	4	6.88
Evaluation strategies												
(109) Both program evaluation and evaluation of learning are included in the evaluation process	3.75	.96	3.89	1.15	4.05	1.02	4.40	.87	4.11	.86	4	4.01
(111) Providers select and/or design tools for evaluating the program and learning	3.48	1.03	3.61	1.17	3.91	1.06	4.36	.94	3.98	1.01	4	6.52
Program implementation												
(114) Providers delineate prerequisite/entry requirements for each offering within the educational program	3.08	1.16	3.66	1.19	3.49	1.14	3.84	1.05	3.54	1.05	4	4.26
(116) Providers establish a time schedule of offerings in the educational program	4.06	.91	4.01	1.00	4.07	.96	4.54	.68	4.47	.85	4	8.58
(117) Program implementation is consistent with the instructional objectives, curriculum and format selected for the program	3.91	.77	3.98	.93	4.11	.87	4.50	.65	4.37	.59	4	9.17

Table 37 —— Summary of significant differences across hospital size for frequency of occurrence of program characteristics — cont'd

Program characteristics	<100 N = 70		100-199 N = 60		200-299 N = 74		300-399 N = 48		400+ N = 72		DF	F*
	X	SD	X	SD	X	SD	X	SD	X	SD		
(118) Program implementation is consistent with the plan for program initiation and the established administrative framework for critical care educational programs	3.75	.77	3.84	.96	3.91	.94	4.25	.75	4.15	.75	4	5.48
Program evaluation												
(136) Critical care instructors participate in program evaluation	3.92	.89	3.98	1.04	4.14	1.01	4.36	.76	4.51	.76	4	4.35
(154) Providers incorporate both formative and summative evaluations of the program	3.10	1.18	3.23	1.14	3.21	1.22	3.88	.91	3.65	1.04	4	6.43
(155) Providers periodically revise programs based on the data contained in the evaluative records	3.72	.88	3.77	.87	4.06	.82	4.23	.70	4.18	.85	4	7.34

The 400+ bed hospital respondents differed significantly from the <200 bed size hospitals on the availability of sufficient reference material for providers (57).

Only the 300-399 to 400+ bed hospital comparison was found not to be significantly different in the availability of clinical experiences to meet the instructional objectives related to nursing practice (66). Respondents from all other categories of hospital sizes differed significantly from each other on their ratings.

Respondents from 100-199 bed hospitals differed significantly from all categories of hospital size greater than 199 on the frequency with which priorities are established among learning needs (76).

The frequency of use of prior program evaluations (86) for determining learning needs was rated as higher in frequency of occurrence by respondents from 300+ bed hospitals than by respondents from either the fewer than 100 or 100-199 bed hospitals. The following five program characteristics from the program goals and objectives category had mean scores by category of hospital size that differed significantly:

(93) Program goals reflect the established priority of learning needs.

(94) Instructional objectives are consistent with and further define the program goals.

(95) Instructional objectives identify the cognitive, psychomotor, and/or affective behaviors of the learner.

(97) Instructional objectives include clearly stated and measurable performance expectations of learners.

(98) Content of the curriculum is selected and leveled to facilitate learner attainment of the instructional objectives.

Respondents from 100-199 bed hospitals differed from those from the 200-299 through the 400+ bed hospitals on program goals reflecting the priority of learning needs (93). The 100-199 bed hospital respondents rated #93 as less frequently occurring when compared to the larger-sized hospitals. The remaining program characteristics present statistically significant differences between fewer than 100 beds and 300-399 and 400+ bed hospitals. In addition the larger the hospital, the greater the frequency of occurrence of instructional objectives being consistent with program goals (94).

Two program characteristics from the evaluation strategy category had mean ratings of frequency of occurrence that differed significantly across hospital sizes. Respondents from the 300-399 bed hospitals differed from respondents in the fewer than 100 bed hospital category on the frequency with which the evaluations of programs and learning are included in the evaluation process (109). The 400+ bed hospital respondents were significantly different from those from fewer than 100 beds hospitals on the extent to which providers select and/or design tools for evaluating the program and learning (111), delineate prerequisite/entry requirements for each offering within the program (114) and establish a time schedule of educational offerings (116). Likewise, program implementation is consistent with instructional objectives (117) and the plan for program initiation and established administrative frameworks for critical care education (118) were rated as more frequently occurring by the 400+ bed hospital respondents as compared to those from fewer than 100 beds hospitals.

Three program evaluation characteristics had mean scores that varied significantly by hospital size (136, 154, 155). The ratings of the frequency of occurrence of these characteristics were such that respondents from the 300-399 and 400+ bed hospitals differed significantly from those from the fewer than 100 beds hospitals. Critical care instructors from larger hospitals more frequently participate in program evaluations (136). The larger-sized hospital respondents more frequently incorporated formative and summative evaluations into programs (154) than did all other respondents. With regard to the revision of programs based on data contained in the evaluative records (155), the 100-199 bed hospital respondents rated it significantly lower than did the 300-399 and 400+ bed hospital respondents.

The ratings of usefulness of program characteristics by size of the respondent hospital are presented in Table 38.

Respondents from the 300-399 bed hospitals rated the usefulness of the documentation of program evaluation (15) higher than did respondents from the fewer than 100 beds hospitals. The availability (64) of storage space was rated more useful by the 400+ bed hospital respondents compared to those from the fewer than 100 beds hospitals. The availability of clinical experiences to meet instructional objectives (66)

Table 38 —— Summary of significant differences across hospital size
for usefulness of program characteristics

Program characteristics	<100 N = 70		100-199 N = 60		200-299 N = 74		300-399 N = 48		400+ N = 72		DF	F*
	X	SD	X	SD	X	SD	X	SD	X	SD		
Program elements												
(15) Documentation of program evaluation	2.97	.77	3.18	.82	3.39	.81	3.47	.65	3.36	.79	4	4.78
Environmental resources												
(64) Storage space is available for material resources and educational records	2.94	.81	2.98	.99	3.25	.92	3.25	.89	3.42	.74	4	4.26
(66) Clinical experiences are available to meet the instructional objectives related to nursing practice	3.40	.74	3.25	.89	3.56	.67	3.54	.66	3.71	.57	4	4.12
Assessment of learning needs												
(76) Providers establish priorities among learning needs relative to the philosophy and goals of the program and available resources	3.34	.67	3.18	.92	3.46	.63	3.34	.70	3.58	.61	4	3.91
Program goals and objectives												
(94) Instructional objectives are consistent with and further define the program goals	3.36	.67	3.20	.73	3.60	.52	3.63	.57	3.60	.60	4	6.87
(95) Instructional objectives identify the cognitive, psychomotor, and/or affective behavior the learner will demonstrate following program participation	3.16	.74	3.30	.69	3.44	.60	3.58	.61	3.49	.69	4	4.45
(97) Instructional objectives include clearly stated and measurable performance expectations of learners	3.37	.66	3.37	.73	3.60	.59	3.63	.53	3.63	.59	4	4.10
Program formats												
(105) Application of principles of adult education	3.36	.69	3.33	.72	3.58	.57	3.41	.65	3.62	.59	4	4.14
Evaluation strategy												
(109) Both program evaluation and evaluation of learning are included in the evaluation process	3.24	.73	3.33	.82	3.56	.60	3.58	.61	3.63	.64	4	5.94
(110) Providers develop a strategy to evaluate application of learning to critical care nursing practice	3.05	.75	3.07	.90	3.55	.65	3.40	.80	3.55	.67	4	7.48

*All significant at P ≤ .01
Usefulness rating scale:

0 = Does not apply	2 = Moderately useful	4 = Extremely useful
1 = Not useful	3 = Quite useful	

Continued.

Table 38 ── Summary of significant differences across hospital size
for usefulness of program characteristics — cont'd

Program characteristics	<100 N = 70		100-199 N = 60		200-299 N = 74		300-399 N = 48		400+ N = 72		DF	F*
	X	SD	X	SD	X	SD	X	SD	X	SD		
Evaluation strategy — cont'd												
(111) Providers select and/or design tools for evaluating the program and learning	3.07	.71	3.17	.87	3.53	.66	3.57	.58	3.62	.57	4	10.07
(112) Providers select and validate tools which contain the criteria to be used during the evaluation process	2.92	.74	3.03	.93	3.38	.78	3.36	.71	3.44	.65	4	6.16
Program implementation												
(114) Providers delineate prerequisite/entry requirements for each offering within the educational program	2.74	.86	3.33	.83	3.22	.83	3.09	.80	3.28	.86	4	3.56
(116) Providers establish a time schedule of offerings in the educational program	3.29	.70	3.50	.72	3.47	.70	3.47	.66	3.70	.55	4	4.37
(117) Program implementation is consistent with the instructional objectives, curriculum and format selected for the program	3.33	.73	3.62	.59	3.50	.72	3.54	.54	3.69	.52	4	3.97
(118) Program implementation is consistent with the plan for program initiation and the established administrative framework for critical care educational programs	3.15	.74	3.42	.61	3.29	.84	3.45	.59	3.65	.51	4	5.62
Program evaluation												
(136) Critical care instructors participate in program evaluation	3.31	.72	3.52	.65	3.54	.64	3.56	.54	3.75	.46	4	3.54
(154) Providers incorporate both formative and summative evaluations of the program	2.92	.93	3.00	.98	3.00	.83	3.30	.68	3.25	.76	4	4.38

was rated by the 400+ bed hospital respondents as more useful than by those from the 100-199 bed hospitals. Respondents from 400+ bed hospitals indicated that establishing priorities among learning needs (76) was more useful than did respondents from hospitals with 100-199 beds.

Respondents from hospitals with more than 200 beds rated the usefulness of instructional objectives being consistent with program goals (94) significantly higher than respondents from 100-199 bed hospitals. Larger hospitals (400+ beds) saw greater usefulness of instructional objectives stating measurable performance expectations of learners (97) as well as identifying the cognitive, psychomotor and affective behavior of learners (95) than did respondents from the 100-199 bed hospitals.

Four evaluation strategy program characteristics were rated in terms of their usefulness. All four were found to be significantly different across categories of hospital size. The 400+ bed hospital respondents had significantly higher ratings of usefulness for the inclusion of program and learning evaluation (109), the development of strategies to evaluate the application of learning to critical care nursing practice (110), the selection of tools for evaluating program and learning (111) and the validation of evaluative tools (112) than did those from the fewer than 100 beds and the 100-199 bed hospitals.

Respondents from hospitals with 400+ beds indicated that they saw the usefulness of providers delineating requirements for each offering (114) and the establishment of a schedule of offerings (116) as higher than respondents from the fewer than 100 beds hospitals. Again, respondents from larger hospitals (400+ beds) see greater usefulness in implementing programs consistent with administrative frameworks (118) and instructional objectives than respondents from hospitals with fewer than 100 beds.

Larger hospital respondents (400+ beds) see greater usefulness in critical care instructors participating in program evaluation than do respondents from fewer than 100 beds hospitals. The judged usefulness of providers incorporating both formative and summative evaluations of programs was significantly higher for the 300-399 bed hospital respondents in comparison to the fewer than 100 bed facility respondents.

Tables 39 and 40 present a summary of those mean differences across categories of hospital size on three program characteristics. Table 39 presents the difference for the frequency with which program characteristics are evaluated by providers and Table 40 reports the same variables evaluated by learners.

In both tables respondents from the larger hospitals (300-399 and 400+ beds) indicated that both providers and learners more frequently evaluate the effectiveness of instructors (148), the quality of instruction (149), and the impact of the learning environment in facilitating learning (150) than do those from hospitals with fewer than 200 beds.

Table 41 presents the mean differences across hospital sizes on the selection criteria for critical care nursing instructors (38). On a four-point scale (1 = not very much, 2 = moderately, 3 = quite, 4 = extremely), the respondents from fewer than 100 beds hospitals provided ratings significantly lower than did respondents from the 300-399 and 400+ beds hospitals on the consistency of the selection criteria for critical care nursing instructors and program goals.

Table 39 ___ Summary of significant differences across hospital size
by frequency of providers

Program characteristics	<100 N = 70		100-199 N = 60		200-299 N = 74		300-399 N = 48		400+ N = 72		DF	F*
	X	SD	X	SD	X	SD	X	SD	X	SD		
Program evaluation												
(148) Effectiveness of instructors	3.75	.91	3.78	.99	4.09	.99	4.39	.64	4.25	.96	4	4.69
(149) Quality of instruction	3.78	.80	3.87	.98	4.09	.90	4.43	.65	4.29	.94	4	5.19
(150) Impact of learning environment in facilitating learning	3.59	1.07	3.57	1.01	3.90	1.06	4.23	.76	3.95	1.08	4	4.92

*All significant at P ≤ .01
Frequency rating scale:
0 = Not applicable   2 = Seldom   4 = Frequently
1 = Never   3 = Sometimes   5 = Always

Table 40 ___ Summary of significant differences across hospital size
by frequency of learners

Program characteristics	<100 N = 70		100-199 N = 60		200-299 N = 74		300-399 N = 48		400+ N = 72		DF	F*
	X	SD	X	SD	X	SD	X	SD	X	SD		
(148) Effectiveness of instructors	3.71	1.00	3.78	1.03	4.17	.81	4.34	.76	4.45	.69	4	8.71
(149) Quality of instruction	3.72	.96	3.78	1.01	4.17	.83	4.28	.80	4.40	.89	4	6.74
(150) Impact of learning environment in facilitating learning	3.45	1.16	3.40	1.07	3.81	1.02	4.04	1.03	3.97	1.12	4	5.11

*All significant at P ≤ .01
Frequency rating scale:
0 = Not applicable   2 = Seldom   4 = Frequently
1 = Never   3 = Sometimes   5 = Always

Table 41 ___ Mean differences across hospital size on selection criteria
for critical care nursing instructors

Program characteristics	<100 N = 70		100-199 N = 60		200-299 N = 74		300-399 N = 48		400+ N = 72		DF	F*
	X	SD	X	SD	X	SD	X	SD	X	SD		
Human resources												
(38) Are the existing selection criteria for critical care nursing instructors consistent with program goals?	2.38	.87	2.70	.96	2.84	.92	2.97	.81	3.03	.92	4	6.42

*All significant at P ≤ .01
1 = Not very much   3 = Quite
2 = Moderately   4 = Extremely

Table 42 ___ Frequency distribution of respondent-reported number of critical care instructors (N = 634)

No. of instructors	Frequency	%
1	289	51.8
2	159	28.5
3	59	10.6
4	24	4.3
5	6	1.1
6	9	1.6
7	4	.7
8	4	.7
9	0	0
10	2	.4
12	1	.2
15	1	.2
TOTAL	634	100.0

Mean	1.68
Standard deviation	1.55
Median	1.00
Range	15.00

Additional survey questions. In addition to statements that were considered to be descriptive of critical care nursing education programs (program characteristics), there were questions asked of respondents that would provide information specifically about selected aspects of human and financial resources and program formats.

Respondents were asked to indicate the number of critical care instructors in their setting. Table 42 is a statistical summary of those responses.

Based on six hundred thirty-four respondents, a range of one to fifteen instructors was reported with a mean of 1.68. It is possible that there could be a greater range in the number of instructors, but the structure of the survey form allowed space for only fifteen instructors.

Table 43 presents a distribution of the number of instructors by the size of the respondents' hospitals. The mean number of reported instructors is 2.39 for the 400+ bed hospital while 1.47 for the fewer than 100 beds hospital. As would be expected, the larger the hospital, the greater the number of instructors.

Respondents were asked to list and provide information about each instructor's highest degree, number of hours of orientation to position as instructor, average number of hours of continuing education per year, number of academic courses in education and the number of courses in clinical specialty. The following information is an analysis of responses to these questions.

Highest degree: Respondents reported on a total of one thousand sixty-six instructors and reported their degree levels as presented in Table 44.

Table 43 ___ Number of reported critical care instructors by size of hospital

No. of instructors	Size of hospital (beds)				
	<100	100-199	200-299	300-399	400+
1	62.1	51.5	62.0	58.9	34.9
2	28.8	27.9	25.3	19.6	28.8
3	9.1	13.2	3.8	10.7	18.1
4		4.4	5.1	3.6	10.8
5				1.8	1.2
6		2.9	1.3		1.2
7				1.8	2.4
8			1.3		2.4
9					
10				1.8	
11					
12				1.8	
13					
14					
15			1.3		
Mean	1.47	1.82	1.81	2.05	2.39
Standard deviation	.66	1.13	1.91	2.11	1.61
Median	1.00	1.00	1.00	1.00	2.00
Range	2.00	5.00	14.00	11.00	7.00

Respondents to the survey form indicated that the largest percentage of instructors across settings have bachelor's degrees (43%) followed by those with master's degrees (26%).

Hours of Orientation: The survey requested that respondents indicate the number of hours of orientation to the position as instructor. The mean number of hours indicated by respondents was 58.92 hours, with a standard deviation of 88.92, and a median of 36.5 hours. The number of hours of orientation ranged from zero (0) to 960 hours. Out of 834 instructors reported on, twenty-two percent (22%) of the instructors had zero (0) hours of orientation.

Hours of Continuing Education: When asked to indicate the average number of hours of continuing education per year for each instructor, respondents reported a range of zero (0) to five hundred (500) hours per year. The mean number of hours was 49.15 with a standard deviation of 69.73 and a median of 35 hours of continuing education per year.

Number of Academic Education Courses: Respondents provided the number of academic courses in education taken by instructors. Table 45 presents the frequency of the number of courses taken by instructors.

The mean number of academic courses in education reported for critical care instructors was 3.95 with a standard deviation of 10.59. The median number of academic courses in education was 1.00. Three hundred six instructors were reported as not having any academic courses in education. This represents forty percent (40%) of all instructors reported on by respondents.

Table 44 —— Highest degree levels of instructors at respondents' practice setting

Value	Degree	N	%
1	Diploma	210	20
2	Associate	111	10
3	Bachelor's	458	43
4	Master's	282	26
5	Doctorate	5	1
	TOTAL	1066	100

Table 45 —— Frequency distribution of respondent-reported number of academic course in education (N = 772)

No. Courses	Frequency	%
0	306	40
1	102	13
2	106	14
3	56	7
4	64	8
5	29	4
6	27	3
7	1	0
8	9	1
9	2	0
10	22	3
10+	48	6
TOTAL	772	100

Number of Courses in Clinical Specialty: Respondents reported that an average of 6.74 courses were taken by instructors in their clinical specialty with a computed standard deviation of 12.04. The number of courses ranged from zero (0), approximately nineteen percent (19%) of instructors, to eighty (80). The median number of courses in clinical specialty was 3.00. Seven hundred fifteen (N = 715) instructors were reported on by respondents.

Table 46 summarizes the means and standard deviations for each of the instructor characteristics reported on by survey respondents. Also contained in Table 46 are the means and standard deviations for the reported number of other health care professionals who provide critical care education.

Respondents reported that an average of 2.23 non-critical-care nurses and 5.61 physicians are involved in the education of critical care nurses. Other health care providers account for an average of 2.81 educators in critical care educational programs.

Reported previously in the program characteristics section of this report was the percent of instructors meeting the nursing practice standards of the critical care

Table 46 ___ Summary of means, standard deviations, and medians for reported instructor educational backgrounds and number of other health care professionals providing education

	N	Mean	S.D.	Median
Instructor's:				
Highest Degree	1066	2.79	1.07	3
No. Hrs. Orient.	834	58.92	88.92	36.5
Avg. No. Hrs. CE/Yr	913	49.15	69.73	35
No. Acad. Ed. Courses	772	3.95	10.59	1
No. Clin. Spec. Courses	715	6.74	12.04	3
Other Health Care Providers:				
Non-critical-care nurses		2.23	3.62	1
Physicians		5.61	6.16	4
Others		2.81	3.83	2

Table 47 ___ Percent of clinical nursing instructors meeting practice standards and demonstrating competence in critical care nursing

Clinical nursing instructor	Mean	S.D.	Median
% meeting nursing standards	87.56	28.72	100
% demonstrating competence	91.15	24.17	100

unit in their area of teaching assignment (36) and the percent who demonstrate competence in the application of nursing and scientific concepts and principles to the care of the critically ill patient (37) broken down by the key respondent variables. Table 47 presents the overall summary of these percentages.

As reported previously there were significant differences between the mean ratings for these two variables (Tables 21, 28 and 33) across categories of key variables. Overall the mean percentage of instructors meeting the nursing practice standards is 87.56% with a median of 100%. Seventy-six percent (76.0%) of the respondents indicated that 100% of the instructors meet these standards while six percent (6.3%) stated that none of the instructors meets the standard.

The percent of instructors who demonstrate competence in the application of nursing and scientific concepts and principles to care of the critically ill patient as rated by survey respondents is 91.15%. The median response was 100%. Seventy-nine percent (79.2%) indicated that 100% of the clinical nursing instructors demonstrated competence. Four percent (4.3%) stated that none of the instructors demonstrated competence in the application of nursing principles to the care of the critically ill patient.

Respondents were asked to provide the average ratio of instructors to learners for classroom (39) and clinical (40) instructors. Table 48 summarizes the means and standard deviations and establishes these ratios.

Table 48 ___ Ratio of instructors to learners for classroom and clinical settings

Type of setting	Instructor		Learner	
	Mean	S.D.	Mean	S.D.
Classroom	1.28	1.63	13.05	10.00
Clinical	1.16	1.03	7.26	13.57

Table 49 ___ Frequency of rank orderings of instructional formats

Rank order	Instructional formats			
	Self-instruction	Lecture	Workshop	Group discussion
1	32	171	327	61
2	44	229	175	150
3	108	151	70	265
4	384	48	31	123

Table 50 ___ Respondent ratings of the number and sufficiency of support personnel (N = 522)

Type of personnel	Number			Sufficiency		
	Mean	S.D.	Med.	Mean	S.D.	Med.
Secretarial staff	1.31	.89	1	2.40	1.11	2
Audiovisual staff	1.24	1.25	1	2.34	1.17	2
Maintenance staff	2.13	2.37	1	2.56	1.14	3
Biomedical engineering	1.90	1.72	1	2.73	1.12	3
Other	2.13	2.75	1	—	—	—*

*Only 55 valid cases.

The ratio of the medians for the classroom instructor-learner ratio is 1:10 and for the clinical instructors the ratio is 1:2.

Respondents were asked to provide a rank ordering of instructional formats based on their judgment of participant preference (1 = most preferred). Table 49 presents the frequency of respondent rankings by type of instructional format.

The instructional format ranked first by most respondents was that of workshops (N = 327). Lecture format was the most frequent second choice (N = 229) followed by group discussion (N = 265). The least preferable instructional format was self-instruction (N = 384).

In addition to gathering information from respondents on instructors in their setting, questions were asked about the support personnel available to facilitate attainment of critical care nursing education program goals. Table 50 summarizes the mean ratings on a four-point scale (1 = insufficient, 2 = somewhat sufficient, 3 = moderately sufficient, 4 = completely sufficient) of the sufficiency of support personnel.

Table 51 —— Sources of financial support for critical care education by type of setting (N = 637)

Sources of support	Primary		Secondary	
	Freq.	%	Freq.	%
If academic setting				
Participant-supported	43	6.8	31	4.9
Employer-supported (nongovernment)	42	6.6	21	3.3
Government	15	2.4	7	1.1
If private continuing education setting				
Participant-supported	55	8.6	29	4.6
Employer-supported (nongovernment)	51	8.0	31	4.9
Government	5	.8	5	.8
If hospital-based setting				
Participant-supported	154	24.2	299	46.9
Employer-supported	456	71.6	129	20.3
Government	53	8.3	37	5.8

The mean rating of the sufficiency of the number of support personnel ranges from a low of 1.24 for audiovisual staff to a high of 2.13 for maintenance and other support staff. The median (Med.) rating of the sufficiency of the number of support staff is one (insufficient) for each category of personnel. The ratings of actual sufficiency of staff has a low mean of 2.34 for audiovisual staff and a high mean of 2.73 for the biomedical engineering staff. The median rating of staff sufficiency is two (somewhat sufficient) for both secretarial and audiovisual staff while the median ratings for maintenance and biomedical engineering staff is three (moderately sufficient).

Respondents were asked to indicate the primary and, if appropriate, secondary sources of financial support as they applied to their setting. Table 51 presents the frequency and percentage of primary and secondary sources of financial support.

The most frequently indicated source of primary support for critical care education is employer-supported programs in hospital-based settings. Seventy-two percent (71.6%) of the respondents saw this as the primary source of support. The indicated secondary source of financial support in the hospital setting is participants (46.9%). Given that (1) the instructions in the survey form requested only one response to this question and the fact that more than 637 responses were recorded and (2) the data presented in Table 1 indicates a small response from academic settings, one questions the data reported in the academic and private continuing education categories in Table 51. A recognition that the respondents are primarily from community-based hospitals leads one to interpret only the hospital-based data in Table 51.

—————— **Summary and Discussion**

The primary objective of this study was to characterize the status of critical care nursing education in the United States. A second study objective was to establish baseline data regarding critical care nursing education for later use in appraising the impact of the AACN Education Standards for Critical Care Nursing. Statements descriptive of programmatic educational activities were used to characterize critical care nursing education programs. In addition demographic data concerning critical care educators were also compiled and analyzed. Data related to the characterization of respondents and program characteristics were analyzed and presented in the results section of this report under two headings: (1) Respondent Characteristics and (2) Program Characteristics.

Respondent characteristics. Those providing critical care nursing (CCN) education can be characterized as female from the 30-39 years of age category. Younger CCN educators tend to have higher degrees. More than sixty-five percent (65%) hold bachelor's and master's degrees. More than ninety percent (90%) hold the designation of CCRN.

Those respondents who classified themselves as administrative (director of critical care nursing, head nurse, supervisor) tend to be slightly older than the educators (director of critical care education, critical care instructor) or clinicians (staff nurse, clinical nurse specialist) and have more associate degrees and diplomas than bachelor's and master's degrees. The administration personnel involved in critical care nursing education tend to be slightly more prevalent in the community hospital environment as compared to educators. This is consistent with the finding that administrative personnel are more actively involved in educational activities within the rural settings and less involved in the suburban and urban settings. Administrators, educators, and clinicians are all predominantly from the 30-39 years of age category.

The administrative personnel tend to have more experience in critical care nursing education and have the same amount of critical care nursing experience as do the educators. The educators tend to come into critical care education later than the administrators. The fact that educators have higher degree levels may account for their fewer years of critical care nursing education experience. The clinical nurse specialists tend to have fewer years of critical care nursing education experience, but their levels of nursing experience are comparable to those of the administrators.

Within the 6-15 years of critical care nursing experience category, there are more bachelor's and master's degrees. As one examines the higher experience levels, there are no differences in degrees obtained and that same relationship holds as well for the lower levels of experience.

As one would expect, those with higher levels of critical care nursing experience tend to be older. The majority of CCN education providers have between 2 and 10 years of experience and are between 30 and 39 years of age. The for-profit hospitals with CCN education programs tend to have staff with more experience in critical care nursing than the nonprofit hospitals.

Approximately eighty percent (80%) of the CCN education providers are from community hospitals. The most frequent degree is the bachelor's followed by the diploma. The community hospitals that are providing for CCN educational programs tend to be evenly distributed between rural, suburban and urban areas. These hospitals also tend to vary greatly in size from 50 to 400+ beds. The military hospitals that house CCN education programs tend to be somewhat larger than the community

Table 52 — Number of significant frequency and usefulness rating comparisons

	1-16 Program elements		17-46 Human resources		47-52 Financial resources		53-58 Material resources		59-66 Environmental resources		67-78 Assessment of learning needs		79-87 Data gathering	
	F	U	F	U	F	U	F	U	F	U	F	U	F	U
Area of practice	7 13		36 37 38				53 55 57	55	66 66	64	68 75		79 81 86	86
Subtotal	0	2	3	0	0	0	3	1	1	2	2	0	3	1
Hospital size		15	38		0	0	57			64 65 66	75 76	76	86	
Subtotal	0	1	1	0	0	0	1	0	0	3	2	1	1	0
Location		15	30				57 58 58	53 54	66	64 66	72	67 72 73	79	
Subtotal	0	1	1	0	0	0	2	3	1	2	1	3	1	0

F = frequency, U = usefulness

by grouping of program characteristics and six key demographic variables

88-92 Resources to achieve goals		93-101 Program goals and objectives		102-108 Program format		109-112 Evaluation strategies		113-133 Program implementation		134-155 Program evaluation		Total	
F	U	F	U	F	U	F	U	F	U	F	U	F	U
91		93	94	102	105	110	109	114	117	136	136		
		94	95	103		111	110	116	123	139			
		95	97	104		112	111	117	126	141			
		96	98	105				118		143			
		97	99					120		144(P)			
		98						121		145(P)			
		99						122		146(P)			
		100						123		148(P)			
		101						125		148(L)			
								126		149(P)			
										149(L)			
										150(P)			
										150(L)			
										152			
										154			
										155			
1	0	9	5	4	1	3	3	10	3	16	1	55	19
F	U	F	U	F	U	F	U	F	U	F	U		
		93	94		105	109	109	114	114	136	136		
		94	95			111	110	116	116	154	154		
		95	97				111	117	117	155	155		
		96					112	118	118	148(P)			
		97								148(L)			
		98								149(P)			
		99								149(L)			
										150(P)			
										150(L)			
0	0	7	3	0	1	2	4	4	4	9	3	27	20
F	U	F	U	F	U	F	U	F	U	F	U		
		93	93		106		110	113	116	136	136		
		94	94				111	117	117	144(P)	139		
		95	95				112	120	118	145(P)	141		
		97	96							148(P)	151		
			97							148(L)	152		
			98							149(P)	153		
			99							149(L)	154		
										150(L)	155		
										154			
										155			
0	0	4	7	0	1	0	3	3	3	10	8	23	31

(P) = education providers, (L) = learners   *Continued.*

Table 52 — Number of significant frequency and usefulness rating comparisons

	1-16 Program elements		17-46 Human resources		47-52 Financial resources		53-58 Material resources		59-66 Environmental resources		67-78 Assessment of learning needs		79-87 Data gathering	
	F	U	F	U	F	U	F	U	F	U	F	U	F	U
Years CC Nsg. Exper		9					58							
Subtotal	0	1	0	0	0	0	1	0	0	0	0	0	0	0
Age			36 37											
Subtotal	0	0	2	0	0	0	0	0	0	0	0	0	0	0
Years CC ED Exper										59 60 61 62 65	72			80
Subtotal	0	0	0	0	0	0	0	0	0	5	1	0	0	1

Table 53 — Number of different items by program characteristic

	1-16 Program elements		17-46 Human resources		47-52 Financial resources		53-58 Material resources		59-66 Environmental resources		67-78 Assessment of learning needs		79-87 Data gathering	
	F	U	F	U	F	U	F	U	F	U	F	U	F	U
N	0	4	4	0	0	0	4	4	1	7	4	4	3	2
%	0	25	13	0	0	0	67	67	14	100	34	34	33	22

F = frequency, U = usefulness

hospitals but not as large as the university hospitals. The university hospitals that have CCN educational programs are primarily the 400+ bed facilities. These facilities primarily have CCN education providers who have bachelor's or master's degrees. The primary source of support for critical care nursing education activities (70%) comes from the hospitals. The secondary source of support is the participant.

The average number of critical care nursing education instructors is reported as 1.68 or approximately two instructors per setting. The majority of these instructors hold bachelor's (38%) and master's (26%) degrees. Instructors who are given an orientation are provided with approximately sixty hours of orientation. Approximately twenty percent of CCN education instructors are not given any type of orientation.

by grouping of program characteristics and six key demographic variables — cont'd

88-92 Resources to achieve goals		93-101 Program goals and objectives		102-108 Program format		109-112 Evaluation strategies		113-133 Program implementation		134-155 Program evaluation		Total	
F	U	F	U	F	U	F	U	F	U	F	U	F	U
		98	98					116	116 117	116	148(L)		
0	0	1	1	0	0	0	0	1	2	0	1	3	5
F	U	F	U	F	U	F	U	F	U	F	U		
0	0	0	0	0	0	0	0	0	0	0	0	2	0
F	U	F	U 96	F	U	F	U	F	U	F	U		
0	0	0	1	0	0	0	0	0	0	0	0	1	7

88-92 Resources to achieve goals		93-101 Program goals and objectives		102-108 Program format		109-112 Evaluation strategies		113-133 Program implementation		134-155 Program evaluation		Total	
F	U	F	U	F	U	F	U	F	U	F	U	F	U
1	0	9	7	4	2	3	4	11	6	16	9	60	49
20	0	100	78	57	28	75	100	52	29	70	39	39	32

These instructors take an average of fifty hours of continuing education per year. Forty percent (40%) have no formal academic courses in education. Those who have courses in education report an average of four. Clinical instructors are reported as having an average of seven courses in their clinical specialty. Close to ninety percent (90%) of the instructors are judged to meet the nursing practice standards of the critical care unit in their area of teaching assignment and demonstrate competence in the application of nursing and scientific concepts and principles to care of the critically ill patient.

The ratio of instructors to learners is very low in programs providing critical care nursing education. For classroom activities the ratio is 1:10 and for clinical work it is 1:2. Workshop formats for instructional activities were judged to be most pre-ferred by program participants followed by lectures and group discussions. The least preferred by the greatest number of raters was the self-instructional format.

Program characteristics. Ninety-eight of the questions provided in the survey required respondents to indicate their ratings of frequency of occurrence and useful-ness of statements that are descriptive of critical care nursing education programs. No effort was made to summarize ratings of frequency of occurrence and usefulness for program characteristics across major groupings. However, in general a review of the overall mean ratings of frequency of occurrence showed that the program character-istics were between a rating of three (3 = sometimes occurring) and four (4 = frequently occurring). The ratings of program elements were somewhat lower indicat-ing that their frequency was somewhere between two (2 = seldom occurring) and three (3 = sometimes occurring). The mean ratings of perceived usefulness by re-spondents was very close to three (3 = quite useful). It is important to note that nearly all of the program characteristics were rated by respondents overall as quite useful to critical care nursing education programs.

In an attempt to better characterize critical care nursing education programs, comparisons of respondent ratings of frequency and usefulness of program character-istics were compared across subgroupings of respondents. These analyses produced one hundred eighty-five statistically significant comparisons between mean ratings. The number of comparisons across groupings of program characteristics by the six key variables is summarized in Table 52. Also included in this table is an indication of whether the specific program characteristic is a rating of frequency or usefulness.

One summary statement that can be made from a review of Table 52 is that the personal characteristics of respondents (years of critical care nursing experience, years of critical care nursing education experience, age) have little to do with ratings of the frequency and usefulness of program characteristic statements. Only seventeen of the one hundred eighty-five significant comparisons were in these categories.

Within the key variables that are institutionally related, there were fewer significant usefulness rating comparisons than frequency of occurrence rating com-parisons. It seems that respondents differ more in their ratings of the frequency of occurrence of program characteristics than in their perceived usefulness. This is probably due in part to the fact that different institutions have different practices. This is also supported by the few significant differences in the program elements, human resources and financial resources categories.

The greatest number of significant differences occurred in the program goals and objectives, evaluation strategy, program implementation and program evaluation categories. It seems that administrators, educators, clinicians and private providers have the greatest differences in their ratings of frequency of occurrence of these program characteristics. Ratings of usefulness of program evaluation tends to be viewed differently more frequently by respondents based on their location.

Table 53 presents a summary of the number of program characteristics that had significant differences across categories of key variables. Specific program charac-teristics that are reported as significant for both frequency and usefulness under one heading are only counted once. This summary table clearly shows that there are greater differences across types of respondents on their ratings of frequency and usefulness by groupings of program characteristics. Critical care nursing educators view their programs quite differently in terms of the program characteristics that are included under the headings of program goals and objectives, evaluation strategy, program implementation and program evaluation.

Limitations. As in any investigation there are limitations that need to be identified to allow for a more deliberate analysis of the findings. The following limitations are recognized in this study:

1. Since there is no listing of critical care nursing education programs, this study first required the identification of those institutions, organizations or individuals providing critical care nursing education. The sources used to initiate this effort as identified in this report may not have been exhaustive.

2. The solicitation of participation in this study was mailed to all hospitals with ICUs and CCUs. Since no specific names were available, the request for participation was addressed to the director of nursing education in care of the hospital. The recipients of the request to participate could have entered their own names or the name of another person at that institution without notifying the other person of the commitment being made. Even though the number of respondents is more than adequate and exceeded what was originally expected, the problems of identifying accurately the respondents could have depressed the response rate.

3. The mailing of the solicitation during the summer months could have been the cause of a lower response rate from academicians and private providers. Both groups may have been more likely to be on vacations.

4. The length of the survey instrument, even though pretested, could have hindered respondents from participating. This could create a biased group of respondents. Given the distribution of respondents as summarized in the results section of this report, however, it seems likely that the group of respondents is reflective of the variety of critical care nursing education programs.

5. The survey instrument did not provide answers to a number of the questions intended for address.

Conclusion. A great deal of data has been summarized on the types of respondents and their descriptions of their critical care nursing education programs. The types of programmatic activities in support of critical care nursing education are extremely institution-specific. Different types of institutions, having program characteristics that differ significantly, with personnel using different titles and breadth of experience, engage in critical care nursing education. It is apparent from this study that varying standards exist for critical care nursing educational activities.